# Asthma
# in Children

Dr Peter van Asperen MD FRACP

Head, Department of Respiratory Medicine
Royal Alexandra Hospital for Children
Sydney, New South Wales

Dr Craig Mellis MB BS MPH FRACP

Director, Clinical Epidemiology Unit and Senior Staff Specialist,
Department of Respiratory Medicine
Royal Alexandra Hospital for Children
Sydney, New South Wales

Jessica Kingsley Publishers
London

First Published by Ashwood House Medical in 1994 as The Chesty Child

First published in the United Kingdom in 1997 by
Jessica Kingsley Publishers Ltd
116 Pentonville Road
London N1 9JB, England
and
1900 Frost Road, Suite 101
Bristol, PA 19007, U S A

Designed and typeset by Q.E.D. Graphic Services
Edited by Janet M Henderson
Illustrations by Julia McLeish

**Library of Congress Cataloging in Publication Data**
A CIP catalogue record for this book is available from the Library of Congress

**British Library Cataloguing in Publication Data**
A CIP catalogue record for this book is available from the British Library

ISBN 1 85302 381 7

Printed and Bound in Great Brita
Athenaeum Press, Gateshead, Ty

# FOREWORD

The 'Chesty child' is a common problem facing parents, particularly during infancy and the early childhood years. Asthma is the commonest cause of recurrent respiratory illness in childhood and, despite improved knowledge about its cause and treatment, it is still misdiagnosed and inappropriately treated in some children.

This book provides the background for understanding the basis of the current approach to asthma management in children. It stresses the importance of co-management – with both the doctor and the parents and/or child being involved in, and responsible for, treatment decisions. It highlights the importance of accurate diagnosis and assessment of severity in ensuring appropriate treatment. The role of regular preventive therapy is emphasised for children with moderate to severe asthma. It addresses many of the questions which parents have when their child is first diagnosed with asthma and provides information on difficult areas, such as the importance of avoiding allergens and the place for alternative therapies. The information provided in this book will increase knowledge about asthma management for parents, children and other health professionals and at the same time, improve the lifestyle for the child with asthma.

The authors are well placed to give their advice. Dr van Asperen heads the Department of Respiratory Medicine in the Royal Alexandra Hospital for children and has a special interest in allergy. Dr Mellis was a former Head of Respiratory Medicine who now directs the Hospital's Clinical Epidemiology Unit. They are both experienced practising paediatricians.

John Yu
Chief Executive
Royal Alexandra Hospital for Children
Sydney, New South Wales

# ACKNOWLEDGMENTS

We would like to thank Karen McKay and Anne-Maree Davis for contributing Chapters 6 and 7 respectively, and for their helpful comments during the development of this book. Special thanks to Angie Mavromihalis and Jackie Cooper for typing and changing the many drafts. We would also like to acknowledge Derek Llewellyn-Jones who encouraged us to write this book and the many asthmatic children and parents who have contributed in their own way to its content. We are also grateful to the following Pharmaceutical Companies: Allen & Hanburys, Astra, Boehringer Ingelheim, Fisons and 3M Riker, for giving us permission to incorporate some of their material into this book.

Finally, we would like to thank our wives, Paula and Jenny and our children Danielle, Jeremy and William, and Duncan, Ian and Scott for their support and encouragement during the evolution of this book.

Peter van Asperen
Craig Mellis

# CONTENTS

# 1

# THE CHESTY CHILD

## INTRODUCTION

Cough and noisy, 'rattly' or wheezy breathing are very common complaints in young children. Indeed, so common that cough in a child is considered normal by some parents. However, cough should *never* be considered normal but rather as a complex and important protective mechanism. Unfortunately, a high percentage of children seem extraordinarily prone to bouts of cough and noisy breathing. Many of these are actually suffering from asthma. The purpose of this chapter is to define cough and wheeze (and other types of noisy breathing) and to explain the mechanism and usual causes of these symptoms. Further, the meaning of the term the 'chesty child' is discussed, together with a guide to symptoms which suggest asthma is the underlying cause of a child's chest symptoms.

## WHAT IS A 'CHESTY CHILD' OR CHESTINESS?

These are loose terms used to describe any child who seems particularly prone to the symptoms of cough, wheeze or a noisy, 'rattly' chest. In approximately half of these children it is due to asthma. In the remainder, it is simply due to recurring bouts of viral respiratory tract infections (colds and flu), which unfortunately in this group of children always seem to result in chest symptoms (a 'chest cold' or acute viral bronchitis). In rare instances, 'chestiness' in a child is due to a serious underlying medical problem, such as bronchiectasis, cystic fibrosis or immune deficiency.

The explanation why some children, who are otherwise normal, are very susceptible to chest infections is unclear. However, since this problem often runs in families, some genetic susceptibility seems at least partly responsible. A similar susceptibility exists in adults with respect to smoking. That is, a proportion of adults develop a persistent cough with sputum (chronic bronchitis) within a short time of taking up smoking. Other adults seem 'immune' to this complication of smoking – at least for many years.

The term 'chestiness' is rather arbitrary. Any child can experience significant chest symptoms, should a serious viral or bacterial infection be contracted, such as: measles, tuberculosis, Mycoplasma pneumoniae, whooping cough or respiratory syncytial virus (RSV bronchiolitis). However, should a normal child suffer from one of these specific, serious infections, it is usually a 'one-off' illness only. Typically, such normal children will have been previously free from chest problems. Further, once they recover from this serious infection, they are not prone to subsequent chest symptoms. By contrast, 'the chesty child' seems vulnerable to chest symptoms from very early childhood to early-mid school years. Typically, each and every minor head cold that comes along provokes the child's chest problem. Since the average pre-school and early school-age child has between six to eight viral respiratory infections per year, this can lead to a very large number of episodes of 'chestiness', particularly during the winter months when viruses are more plentiful.

## THE DEFINITION AND CAUSES OF COUGH

*Cough is defined as the explosive release of air from the chest at high speed for the purpose of removing secretions, or irritants, from the bronchial tree and lungs.*

A cough is very similar to a sneeze. Except that a sneeze has the purpose of removing secretions, or irritants, from the nose. Coughing is only one of a number of ways in which the lungs and airways remain free from excessive secretions. The usual, first-line mechanism is the muco-ciliary escalator. This is a 'moving footway' made up of small hairs (cilia) on the surface of the airways. These cilia continually beat and sweep secretions up from the lower respiratory tract to the throat, where they are then swallowed. Normally, cough is not required, unless the secretions are either excessive in amount, or thicker than normal (infected). Thus, cough should be seen as a 'fail-safe', or 'back-up' mechanism – only brought into play when the muco-ciliary escalator is overloaded. Under these circumstances, the cough will usually be described as: loose, 'fruity' or productive.

This type of cough should be distinguished from throat clearing or 'hawking'. This is due to drawing back secretions from the back of the throat or nose (catarrh or post-nasal drip). This common, unpleasant habit does not have the same significance as a genuine, explosive cough arising from the lower airways/lungs.

The other common trigger for true cough is when the airways are irritated. This can be due to agents which are irritants for all of us, such as potent fumes (high concentrations of chlorine or ammonia) or large amounts of dust or smoke. Alternatively, it can be due to an excessive sensitivity to 'normal' everyday exposures, such as perfumes, the smell of animals (cats or horses), or low concentrations of smoke, dust or fumes. This is particularly likely in children with asthma. Under these circumstances, the cough is generally described as dry, irritative or unproductive. The many possible causes of cough are listed in Table 1.1 and discussed in detail later.

The mechanism for cough is complex and shown in Figures 1.1 and 1.2. Although cough can be triggered voluntarily or suppressed consciously, it is

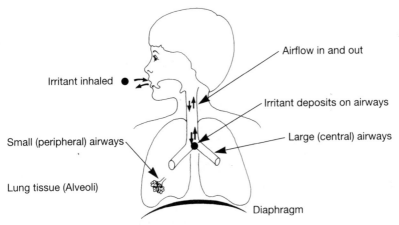

**Figure 1.1**: Normal breathing

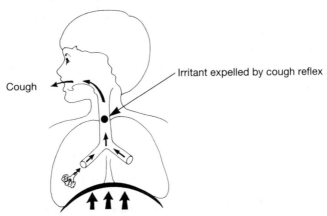

Diaphragm contracts forcing air and irritant out of airways

**Figure 1.2**: Cough after irritant enters airways (The cough reflex)

normally a complex reflex action. This reflex results from stimulation of cough receptors (nerve fibres) in the airways. When stimulated, (either by secretions or irritants), nerve impulses travel to cough centres in the brain stem. The cough centre then co-ordinates a complicated series of muscular activities involving the diaphragm and larynx (voice box). The end result is an explosive, effective cough designed to remove the offending irritant, or the excessive secretions, from the airways.

**Table 1.1:** Causes of cough

| Very common | Less common | Rare |
| --- | --- | --- |
| 1 Asthma | 1 Cigarette smoke | 1 Foreign body inhalation |
| 2 Acute viral bronchitis | 2 Acute bacterial bronchitis<br>Whooping cough<br>Mycoplasma pneumoniae | 2 Pulmonary aspiration<br>3 Tuberculosis<br>4 'Nervous/habit' cough |
| | 3 Bronchiectasis/chronic bronchitis<br>Cystic fibrosis<br>Immune deficiency | |

Causes of cough according to age

1  Infants (age 0-1 year)
Although viral colds and bronchitis can occur in young infants, they are less frequent in this age group because of inborn immunity (derived from their mothers), and less exposure to other young children. Therefore, a persistent or troublesome cough in early infancy is a reason to seek early medical advice. Rare malformations of the airways, lungs and upper gastro-intestinal tract need to be excluded, as do some unusual congenital chest infections which can occur in this age group. The possibility that the baby is inhaling his or her feeds, either during feeding, or shortly after feeding (due to reflux of stomach contents into the throat) may also need to be considered.
In most cases, however, troublesome cough in this age group is the result of a particularly potent virus, called RSV (Respiratory Syncytial Virus). This virus visits our community every winter in epidemic proportions – usually for several months. Unfortunately, there is no available vaccine, and many babies who are infected develop a significant chest illness, called acute viral (RSV) bronchiolitis. This illness causes severe cough, wheeze and breathlessness. Approximately one in 50 babies who develop this illness require admission to hospital because of severe shortness of breath, and many need oxygen for several days, until the illness subsides spontaneously. In some babies

with bronchiolitis, a distressing cough persists for some weeks after all other symptoms have disappeared.

2 Toddlers – pre-schoolers (age 1-4 years)
In this age group, viral infections are rampant! Thus, those children who are prone to chest symptoms with viruses (the 'chesty child'/recurrent acute bronchitis) can expect to suffer repeated bouts, particularly in the winter months. Asthma is also more common in this age group than at any other time in life. Moreover, most young children with asthma will have a 'flare-up' of their asthma symptoms when they get a viral infection. This unfortunate combination spells trouble for these youngsters and their parents. Fortunately however, as immunity to the common viruses develops, with increasing age, the frequency and severity of the chest symptoms will improve – irrespective of whether the cause is asthma or recurrent viral bronchitis. Thus, both these common entities, asthma and recurrent viral bronchitis, become progressively less common once this age period has been passed.
Rarer, but more serious causes of cough in this age group are inhaled foreign bodies (especially peanuts and other nuts) and some of the rare chronic infective lung problems (such as bronchiectasis, as a result of cystic fibrosis or immune deficiency).

3 Primary school children (age 5-12 years)
The usual causes of cough in this age group are acute bronchitis and asthma. Viruses are the most common infections causing bronchitis, although bacterial causes such as whooping cough (Bordetella pertussis) and Mycoplasma pneumoniae can be important when these micro-organisms are epidemic in the community.

4 High school students and adolescents (age 13-18 years)
Although asthma and acute viral bronchitis are still common in this age group, troublesome cough appearing for the first time at this age suggests either an unusual infection (Mycoplasma pneumoniae) or cigarette smoking. A nervous or habit cough ('attention-seeking' cough) is also common in this age group. Typically this cough is loud and 'brassy,' disappears during sleep, and results in considerable secondary gain (especially prolonged school absence).

## THE DEFINITION AND CAUSES OF WHEEZE

*A wheeze is defined as a whistling noise arising from the chest, often accompanied by a sensation of difficulty in breathing. It is usually louder when the child is breathing out.*

This wheezing noise arises because the bronchial tubes through which air moves in and out of the lungs, are narrower than usual. Hence, the air movement is not silent, but turbulent and audible. Narrowing of the airways can be due to a large number of causes. These are broadly classified as obstructing either *small* (peripheral) or *large* (central) airways (Table 1.2). These causes will be discussed in detail below. It is important to understand the very close link between cough and wheeze. Thus, the causes of both are similar; it is common for both symptoms to be present together; and it is also likely that cough can lead to wheeze, and vice versa.

## The causes of wheeze according to age

1    Infants (age 0-1 year)
     In very young infants, the possibility of some *malformation* in either the lungs, airway or chest must be considered a possibility, particularly if the wheezing is severe and associated with marked shortness of breath or poor weight gain. If infants develop breath holding (apnoea) or blue discolouration of the lips associated with wheezing, the condition is extremely severe and demands urgent medical attention. Wheezing due to *asthma* can occur in the first year of life. Generally this wheezing is soft and unassociated with obvious shortness of breath. Infants with asthma usually do not require treatment. Furthermore, their response to anti-asthma therapy is not as good as that seen in older children with typical asthma. By far the commonest cause of wheezing in the first year of life is best considered 'physiologic' wheezing. Infants have smaller airways than older children and the smaller these airways the more likely there is to be a noise associated with breathing. In addition, infants have relatively soft, 'floppy' bronchial tubes. Thus if breathing is forced or hard (with feeding, laughing or crying) then the pressure dynamics within the chest are such that the airways can narrow transiently, during these high-pressure situations. This so-called physiologic wheezing is very common in infancy. It is of no medical significance and disappears as the child becomes older, as the airways grow and their walls become more solid. It has many similarities to the innocent cardiac murmur, a heart murmur which can be heard in many normal children, (particularly at times of fever or heavy exercise) which disappears as they grow.
     During the winter months, if an infant develops an acute 'cold' followed by cough and wheezing, then the likelihood of RSV bronchiolitis (acute viral bronchiolitis) is extremely high. As described previously, this is epidemic in the Australian community each winter, and wheezing is a very common symptom with this infection. The wheeze usually settles over several days and in most infants is not particularly severe, nor does it warrant any specific treatment.

2   Toddlers – pre-schoolers (age 1-4 years)
    Wheezing in this age group is generally due to asthma. These children
    have recurrent episodes of wheeze particularly with viruses (colds/flu).
    Foreign body inhalation is also common in this age group, and peanuts
    (or any other nuts) should *never* be given to these young children.

3   Primary school children (age 5-12 years) and high school  students/
    adolescents (age 13-18 years)
    Recurrent wheezing in these age groups is virtually always due to
    asthma, and there is generally no difficulty making this diagnosis.

## THE DEFINITION OF OTHER FORMS OF NOISY BREATHING

*Stridor* is a loud, 'crowing' sound, heard best when the child is breathing-in
(during inspiration). It is often accompanied by a brassy, barking or 'croupy'
cough and a hoarse voice or cry (laryngitis). It is most commonly heard when
young children have 'viral croup' (viral-laryngo-tracheo-bronchitis), an
acute viral infection of the trachea (wind-pipe) and larynx (voice-box). 'Viral
croup' generally lasts for several days, and it is usually worse at night.

### Table 1.2: Causes of wheeze

(a) Large or central airway obstruction (Larynx. Trachea. Main bronchi)
   **Congenital malformations**
   *Larynx*
   Larynogomalacia – softness or 'floppiness' of tissue in voice box)

   *Trachea and bronchial tree*
   Tracheomalacia or bronchomalacia (abnormally 'floppy' or soft central airways)
   Tracheal or bronchial stenosis (congenital narrowing)
   Vascular ring (e.g. double aortic arch – which 'chokes' the windpipe)

   *Airway or lung cysts/tumours*
   (Large mass in chest which deforms and narrows the central airways)
   **Foreign bodies:**
   Inhaled (laryngeal, tracheal or bronchial)
   Swallowed: (upper oesophagus)

(b) Small or peripheral airway obstruction (bronchi and bronchioles)
   **Asthma**
   Acute viral bronchiolitis
   Especially respiratory syncytial virus (RSV)

   **Familial (early onset) bronchiectasis**
   Cystic fibrosis
   Primary ciliary dyskinesia (immotile cilia syndrome)
   Congenital hypo-gamma-globulinaemia

   **Recurrent pulmonary aspiration**
   Secondary to disorders of swallowing
   Secondary to gastro-oesophageal reflux
   Anatomic communication between gastro-intestinal and respiratory tract.

*A rattle* in the chest is usually due to excessive fluid or secretions in the large, central air passages. The rattle is usually heard both during inspiration and expiration, and may be felt if the hands are placed over the child's chest. It is most commonly heard in very young children during bouts of either viral bronchitis or asthma. Following an effective bout of coughing, the 'rattliness' may temporarily improve, (particularly if viral bronchitis is the cause) as the secretions are cleared (usually swallowed).

*A snuffle* is a noise arising from the nose and is due to narrowing of the nasal passages. This can be the result of either swelling of the lining of the nose or excessive secretions in the nose. It is common with colds/flu and during a bout of hay fever/nasal allergy.

*Snoring* is not unique to adults. It is very common in young children, and is usually the result of large tonsils and adenoids. These enlarged lymphoid tissue masses partly block the flow of air entering the throat and nose, particularly when the child is in deep sleep.

## CLINICAL FEATURES SUGGESTING ASTHMA

Clearly, wheezing may be due to causes other than asthma. However, there are various clinical features, of both the cough and the wheeze, which suggest asthma is the cause.

1  Cough
   In children with asthma, the cough is usually dry and irritating and particularly prominent at night and in the early evening, around dusk. Cough often wakes these children, particularly in the early hours of the morning. The cough is also prominent after exercise – particularly vigorous running.

2  Wheeze
   A history of recurrent, discrete episodes of loud wheezing is highly suggestive of asthma – but not proof. Loud wheezing that comes on after vigorous exercise or during sleep is almost certainly due to asthma. If the wheezing disappears promptly following the inhalation of a bronchodilator agent (Ventolin, Respolin, Bricanyl, Berotec), then asthma is almost certainly the cause.

3  Shortness of breath/difficulty breathing
   Wheezing which is accompanied by 'tightness' in the chest and/or difficulty in breathing, and which comes on particularly at night/early morning, or with exercise, and disappears with a bronchodilator, is almost certainly due to asthma. In asthmatic children it is particularly common for them to wake first thing in the morning and complain of some 'tightness' in the chest and shortness of breath. After they have

been awake for some time, moving around, and eating breakfast, the tightness disappears. Some young children describe this as 'pain' in the chest or 'tummy pain'.

**4**   Family history of allergy (atopy)
If a parent (especially if both), or one of the child's siblings (brother or sister) has asthma, eczema or nasal allergy (hay fever), then lower respiratory symptoms such as cough or wheeze are highly likely to be due to asthma, rather than one of the other causes previously mentioned.

**5**   Personal medical history of allergy (atopy)
If the child with the lower respiratory symptoms (cough and/or wheeze) has a past or present history of eczema or nasal allergy, then again the respiratory symptoms in the chest are almost certainly due to asthma.

**6**   Response to anti-asthma treatment
As mentioned before, if the cough, wheeze or breathing difficulty promptly disappear (within three to five minutes) following the administration of a bronchodilator aerosol, then asthma is very likely the cause. Further, if the use of regular, preventive therapy such as Intal or inhaled corticosteroids (Becotide or Pulmicort) over a period of three to six weeks results in disappearance of the lower respiratory symptoms, then asthma is almost certainly the cause.

**7**   Examination of the child
If the child in question has generalised wheezy noises when the doctor listens to the chest with a stethoscope, asthma will be suspected. Additionally, the doctor will look for evidence of eczema and nasal allergy as mentioned previously, and may administer a bronchodilator aerosol to assess the response three to five minutes after. If the abnormal signs disappear, this confirms the presence of asthma.

**8**   Investigations/diagnostic tests
Tests which indicate the presence of allergy (atopy) are either RAST tests (blood tests) or allergen skin-prick tests. If positive, then asthma is more likely – especially if there are multiple large reactions. Chest X-rays are usually normal in children with asthma, particularly in the interval between acute attacks. Lung function tests (such as peak flow or spirometry), if done between attacks, will also usually be normal in the asthmatic child. If the lung function is abnormal, then it is usual to administer a bronchodilator, and repeat the measurements to see if this reverses the abnormality. If positive, this test, is one of the strongest pieces of evidence to prove asthma. These tests are discussed in more detail in subsequent chapters.

## SUMMARY

- Cough and wheeze are common symptoms in infants and young children.
- Although cough and wheeze are classical features of asthma, other conditions can cause these symptoms, particularly in infancy.
- The age of the child and the features of the cough and wheeze (plus other symptoms) are helpful in determining whether these symptoms are due to asthma – or some other underlying cause.
- Although very common in young children, asthma does have a generally favourable outlook, particularly if the symptoms are infrequent and only associated with viral infection.

# 2

# WHAT IS ASTHMA?

## INTRODUCTION

### Historical perspective

The term asthma was first used by the Greeks around 400 BC to describe varying degrees of breathing difficulty. Thus 'dyspnoea' referred to moderate distress, 'asthma' to more marked distress and 'orthopnoea' to severe distress. To these early Greeks, such as Hippocrates, asthma was considered merely a symptom and it was not until AD 100, in the writings of Aretaeus, that asthma was first considered a disease. He described the spasmodic nature of the disease and its tendency to be provoked by exertion.

Some understanding as to the cause of asthma had to await the Renaissance. In the seventeenth century, a Belgian physician, Jean Van Helmont, himself an asthmatic, described asthma as due to, 'a drawing together of the Bronchi.' Two English physicians, Thomas Willis and Sir John Floyer further expanded this concept. Willis described 'cramps of the moving fibres of the bronchia and of the vessels of the lung, diaphragm and muscles of the breast.' Floyer stated, 'in the asthmatic fit, the muscular fibres of the bronchia and vessels of the lungs are contracted and that produces the wheezing noise, which is most observable in expiration.'

During the eighteenth and nineteenth centuries, further refinements in the understanding of asthma occurred. The recognition of a distinct layer of muscle in the bronchial wall which, when it contracted, constricted the bronchial airways, confirmed the previous suggestions that asthma was due to spasm of the airways. The apparent importance of allergy in provoking asthma led to the classification of asthma as an 'allergic' disease by Samuel Meltzer, a New York physician, in 1910.

### Current concepts of asthma

Asthma may mean different things to different people:
To the child or parent, it will mean an incessant cough, an audible wheeze or a feeling of difficulty in breathing, much in the way the term was used by the ancient Greeks.

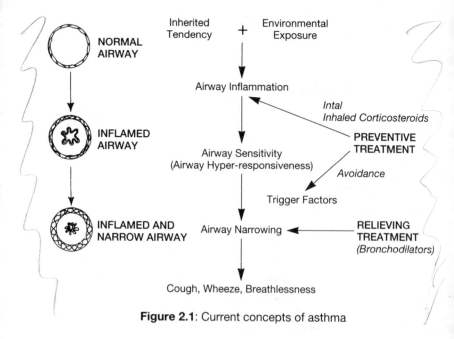

**Figure 2.1**: Current concepts of asthma

To the doctor, it is a disease in which the child presents with recurring episodes of cough, wheeze or breathlessness which respond to treatment with medications which allow the airways to open (bronchodilators).

To the physiologist, asthma is a disease characterised by airways which are more sensitive than normal airways ('hyper-responsive') and are therefore more likely to narrow in response to exposure to a variety of trigger factors.

To the pathologist, asthma is a disease characterised by inflammation of the airways. This appears to result because of an inherited tendency for the airways to become inflamed interacting with environmental factors, which induce the state of airway inflammation. The airway inflammation, in turn, makes the airways more sensitive, resulting in airway narrowing in response to certain triggers. The airway narrowing produces the cough, wheeze or breathlessness seen in the child with asthma.

An understanding of these concepts of asthma is important in compre-hending the basis of the current treatment of asthma. Thus, emphasis in the past has been on treating the symptoms of cough, wheeze and breathlessness with medications which relieved the airway narrowing (bronchodilators). While clearly this symptomatic treatment improved the patient's distress, it had no effect on the underlying inflammation or airway sensitivity, so the patient was likely to develop further episodes of cough and wheeze when re-exposed to certain trigger factors. In fact, recent evidence would suggest that in some situations frequent use of bronchodilator medications may even be making the airways more sensitive. Current emphasis is therefore on *preventive* treatment, either by using medications which reduce airway inflammation and airway sensitivity or by avoiding trigger factors. Thus, episodes of cough and wheeze may be prevented rather than just treated when symptoms arise. The ultimate aim of asthma treatment will be to prevent the onset of airway inflammation, which clearly will depend on a better understanding of those environmental factors which are important in converting an inherited tendency to a disease state.

The remainder of this chapter will explore in more detail these basic concepts of asthma to provide the reader with an insight into the nature of the disease and the rationale for its treatment.

## AIRWAY NARROWING

In order to understand the cause of asthmatic symptoms, it is important to have some background knowledge on the structure and function of the lung. The lung consists of a series of branching tubes (airways or bronchi) which carry air to the air sacs (alveoli). The function of the lung is to exchange oxygen in the air with carbon dioxide from the bloodstream. The oxygen is required for the functioning of all the cells in the body and, as a result of this

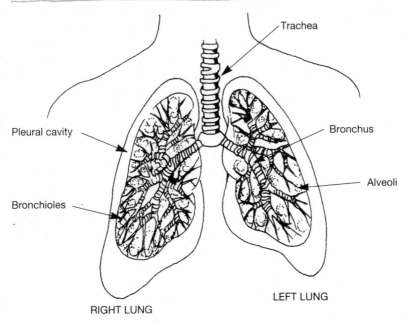

**Figure 2.2**: Anatomy of the lung

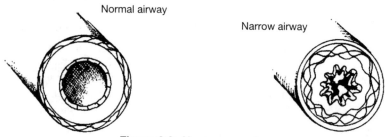

**Figure 2.3**: Airway narrowing

cellular metabolism which requires oxygen, the carbon dioxide which is produced needs to be removed. With each breath, air passes through the nose and/or mouth into the major airways (trachea and major bronchi) and then into the smaller airways and finally the alveoli. Oxygen then diffuses into the bloodstream and carbon dioxide diffuses back into the alveoli and then back up the series of airways into the atmosphere.

Asthma is a disease of the smaller conducting airways in the lung. The normal airway consists of a surface lining of cells (the epithelium), mucus secreting glands which lie under the epithelium, and outside this a layer of muscle surrounding the airway. During an episode of asthma, the muscle contracts, narrowing the airway. There is also swelling of the inner layers of the airway wall and increased mucus production resulting in plugs of mucus in the airway. These three pathological features may occur to varying degrees during an episode of asthma, thus explaining different symptoms. When airway narrowing is severe, breathlessness is likely to be a major feature, while if narrowing is mild, cough may be the only symptom. In some children excessive mucus secretion predominates and a moist cough may be the principal feature. The characteristic 'tight' cough in an asthmatic child might represent the inability to clear mucus from a narrowed airway or reflect irritation of nerve endings in the cellular lining.

This simple model of airway narrowing in asthma assumes that the airway was previously normal. However, we now know that the asthmatic airway is abnormal even between acute episodes of cough and wheeze. As a result, the asthmatic airway reacts to triggers in the manner described above, resulting in airway narrowing – and the typical symptoms of asthma. What makes these airways abnormal is *inflammation*.

## AIRWAY INFLAMMATION AND AIRWAY HYPER-RESPONSIVENESS

Inflammation is the body's normal response to injury or infection and usually results in healing. In some situations, persisting inflammation may result in

**Normal airway**

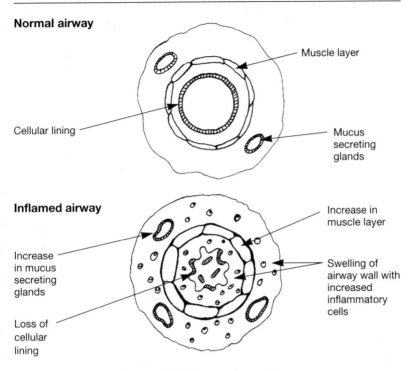

**Figure 2.4**: Airway inflammation

a disease process, for example, rheumatoid arthritis. Inflammatory changes in the airway have long been recognised as part of the acute episode of asthma, manifested by increased mucus secretion and swelling of the lining of the airway – both of which contribute to airway narrowing. More recently, it has been recognised that a state of persisting airway inflammation exists in patients with asthma. Thus, even in asthmatic patients who are completely free of symptoms, the airway remains inflamed. The normal cellular lining is disrupted, the airway wall is swollen and contains various inflammatory cells (eosinophils, neutrophils and mast cells) and there are increased numbers of mucus secreting glands and cells. There is also an increase in the amount of muscle surrounding the airway, which is possibly a result of the abnormal inflammatory process. How this inflammation first appears and why it persists is still not clear, although we now recognise a number of factors which may be important. What is clear, however, is that there are unique features of this persistent airway inflammation, particularly the presence of white blood cells called eosinophils, which are characteristic of the asthmatic patient. Unravelling the events that lead to this state may help us to understand better the cause of asthma.

Another feature that appears to characterise the asthmatic patient is airway hyper-responsiveness. This refers to an increase in the sensitivity of the airways, such that the airway of the asthmatic patient narrows in response to exposure to a variety of trigger factors while the airway of a person without asthma does not. The tendency to wheeze after exercise or after laughing is an example of airway hyper-responsiveness. This hyper-responsiveness can be demonstrated in the laboratory by provoking the airways with certain triggers (exercise, cold air, water, or drugs such as histamine and methacholine). Although airway hyper-responsiveness is not unique to, or universal in, asthmatic subjects, it is a feature which does help us to characterise the patient with asthma. In general, there appears to be a good correlation between the degree of hyper-responsiveness (that is, how sensitive the airways are) and both the severity of asthma symptoms and the outcome of childhood asthma.

What is the relationship between airway inflammation and airway hyper-responsiveness? While the exact mechanism of airway hyper-responsiveness remains unclear, there are a number of potential ways that airway inflammation may contribute to abnormal airway sensitivity. Destruction of the epithelial lining may have a number of effects. It may expose nerve endings which can then be more easily stimulated and result in an increased tendency for the muscle to contract in response to trigger factors. The disruption of the lining cells may also allow various triggers direct access to the muscle. In addition the lining cells contain a factor which inhibits muscle contraction and its loss may make the muscle more likely to narrow the airway. The inflammatory cells in the airway wall secrete various chemicals which may enhance the tendency for the airways to narrow by a variety of mechanisms. It has recently been suggested that the swelling and thickening of the airway wall, resulting from the inflammatory process, may give rise to an exaggerated narrowing of the airway when the muscle contracts normally. Another suggestion is that the muscle itself reacts abnormally, although this has been difficult to prove.

In summary, it appears that the tendency for the airways to narrow in an asthmatic subject is due to airways that are more sensitive than normal. This increased sensitivity may result from the state of persistent airway inflammation which is seen in the airway of the asthmatic patient.

## TRIGGER FACTORS

The term 'trigger factor,' refers to those factors which are known to produce airway narrowing in patients with asthma. In general, the more sensitive the airway, the larger the number of factors likely to provoke airway narrowing, and thus episodes of cough and wheeze. In children at the mild end of the asthma spectrum, only viral infections, such as common colds, are likely to provoke asthma attacks as they are the most potent trigger factor. On the other hand, in children with more severe forms of asthma, many of the trigger factors listed below are likely to provoke wheezing.

While many of the trigger factors simply provoke airway narrowing in the asthmatic subject, some of these factors may also transiently increase airway responsiveness. In particular, viral infections and allergen exposure, are known to increase airway sensitivity for a time, and this is most likely due to inflammatory changes which occur as a result of the exposure. This explains why many children may have a period of persistent symptoms such as night-time cough, following an episode of wheezing. In these situations, an increase in the preventive treatment may help control this increase in airway sensitivity, and thus reduce the symptoms.

Trigger factors which may be important in provoking your child's asthma include:

1    Viral Infections
     Viral infections, such as the common cold, are the most important trigger in childhood and account for up to 50 per cent of acute episodes of wheezing, particularly in the pre-school age group. Children have an average of six to eight viral respiratory infections a year in the first five to six years of life, and if there is any degree of increased airway sensitivity, will probably develop cough and wheeze in association with a least some of these infections. In many pre-school children, viral infections are the only trigger for their asthma giving rise to the pattern of autumn/winter asthma with summers generally free of symptoms.

2    Exercise
     Exercise-induced wheezing as a feature of asthma has been recognised since the times of Aretaeus, around AD100. In fact exercise-induced airway narrowing, as a means of demonstrating the presence of airway hyper-responsiveness, appears to be unique to asthma, while other measures of airway hyper-responsiveness may be seen in other respiratory illnesses. The cause of exercise-induced asthma is thought to be related to the loss of heat and water from the airways during exercise, and thus exercise in which this is likely to be pronounced: for example, running is more likely to provoke wheezing. Swimming is often recommended as a good exercise for asthmatic children because it is less likely to cause wheezing. The degree of exercise-induced asthma, or reduction in the ability to exercise, is a good measure of asthma severity, as it usually reflects the degree of airway sensitivity.

3    Allergies
     Children with asthma often have a tendency to develop allergic reactions to foreign substances, such as foods and airborne particles.

These substances which elicit an allergic response are termed 'allergens'. These reactions are due to the development of a certain type of antibody, called IgE, which when formed, will react with the ingested or inhaled allergen causing an allergic reaction. This reaction is due to the release of a number of chemical substances from cells which contain the IgE antibody on their surface (mast cells). Depending on the site of this reaction, the patient may develop different symptoms: hives or swelling in the skin; vomiting in the gut; sneezing or discharge from the nose or wheezing from the airway. This tendency for people to make IgE antibodies is termed atopy (a Greek word meaning 'strange disease'), and is found more commonly in children with asthma, eczema and allergic nasal problems. These diseases are referred to as *atopic diseases* and often occur together in the atopic child.

Allergic food reactions occur most commonly in the first year or two of life, usually to a limited range of foods – milk, eggs, and peanuts being by far the most common. Reactions due to the presence of the IgE antibody are immediate, occurring within minutes of eating the food and lasting only a few hours. Although allergic food reactions occur in asthmatic children because of the association with atopy, food allergy is not usually a major trigger factor of wheeze. Hives, vomiting, colic and runny nose are more common than wheezing as a manifestation of these immediate food reactions. In addition, many children with these types of food reactions become tolerant to the food after the first year of life. It is often said that asthmatic children should avoid milk because it increases mucus production. There is little evidence to support this suggestion and generally, milk can be tolerated without problem in children with asthma. Reactions to food additives, which do not involve an allergic reaction will be considered later.

Airborne allergens appear to be more important causes of allergic reactions in the airways, as they gain access by direct inhalation. Common sources of these allergens include trees and grasses (pollens), insects (house dust mite, cockroach), moulds (fungi) and pets (cats, dogs, horses). While there has been much work previously on experimental inhalation of these substances, it is only recently that investigators have focused on the likely exposure of these substances to patients in the home setting. While some patients develop obvious immediate symptoms following exposure to these airborne particles, inhaled allergens appear to be relatively uncommon as trigger factors for acute episodes of wheezing. However, low-grade exposure to these allergens may be important in inducing and maintaining the state of increased airway responsiveness.

**4**    Food additives and medications

It is now well recognised that certain food additives and medications can trigger episodes of wheezing through non-allergic mechanisms, often termed sensitivities. These reactions appear more likely to occur in patients with more sensitive airways. In children with persistent asthma, about two-thirds react to the preservative metabisulphite, and about one-quarter to aspirin. Interestingly, removal of the offending substances from the diet is only helpful in improving asthma in a minority of cases, suggesting that while these substances can trigger attacks of asthma, they do *not* alter airway sensitivity.

Metabisulphite is used to preserve foods by preventing oxidation and appears to be the most important of the food additives provoking asthma. In children, it is most likely to trigger asthma when in the liquid form, for example, juices, pickles, salads. It is thought to cause problems by the release of sulphur dioxide which is directly irritant to the airway. Although monosodium glutamate, a flavour enhancer used in cooking, has been documented as a cause of wheezing in adults, it appears to be an uncommon cause of wheezing in asthmatic children. Tartrazine, a yellow food colouring, while often implicated as a cause of wheezing, has never been documented as a cause of asthma in children. Aspirin (acetylsalicylic acid) should be avoided in asthmatic children because of its potential to trigger wheezing. Paracetamol is generally tolerated without a problem. There is little evidence to suggest that avoidance of foods containing natural salicylate is important, even in patients who are known to be sensitive to aspirin.

**5**    Changes in the weather

Parents often relate their child's asthma to sudden changes in weather conditions. These observations have been supported by studies indicating that hospital attendances and admission rates are affected by certain weather changes. The exact mechanism of this association remains unclear but could include release of airborne allergens or irritants or direct effects of climatic conditions on the airways. 'Thunderstorm'-induced asthma has recently been shown to be due to the release of grass pollen allergens, in particles small enough to enter the airways.

**6**    Emotional factors

Emotional triggers can certainly be important in some children with asthma, both by increasing the severity of episodes and also in some situations precipitating episodes. These effects appear to be mediated by the brain, via nerves, which affect the airways. In young children, excitement-induced wheezing may be related more to exercise than to emotional factors.

7    Air pollution
Outdoor air pollution, although much publicised, appears to have a very limited effect on provoking asthma, as pollutants seldom reach concentrations high enough to cause wheezing. In contrast, indoor air pollution, particularly from cigarette smoke, is an important trigger factor for respiratory illness in childhood. Passive smoking, particularly from the mother, has been associated with an increase in asthmatic symptoms and airway sensitivity in the child. In older children and teenagers, active smoking is equally harmful. Other potential sources of indoor air pollution include wood stoves and unflued gas heaters, although these appear much less likely to cause problems when compared with cigarette smoke, because of the relatively low levels of pollutants encountered.

## DEVELOPMENT OF AIRWAY HYPER-RESPONSIVENESS

The induction and maintenance of airway hyper-responsiveness in asthmatic patients is a very complex process, involving both inherited and environmental factors. There remain many unanswered questions. Some recent evidence suggests that all infants may be born with the potential to develop atopy and airway hyper-responsiveness, and that the development of asthma depends more on an inability to lose these tendencies as the infant matures rather than their induction. What seems to be becoming increasingly apparent is that the tendency to develop asthma may be determined very early in life, even *before* birth, and any attempts to prevent its development will need to be made at this early age (*see* Figure 2.5).

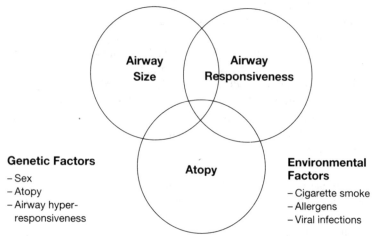

**Figure 2.5**: Determinants of wheeze in childhood

1    Inheritance
The inheritance of asthma is complex but there is a clear indication in many children with asthma of a family tendency to asthma or one of the other atopic diseases. From studies in families of asthmatic children, it appears that there may be separate inherited factors (genes) controlling the tendency for the airways to be hyper-responsive and also the tendency to atopy, that is, the formation of IgE antibodies. The atopic gene appears to be important in determining the severity and outcome of asthma in children. Those children with eczema, nasal allergy and IgE antibodies to many allergens are more likely to have persisting problems than those whose asthma appears related only to viral infections. The recent suggestion that the atopic gene has been identified may help in our understanding of the mechanisms involved in the development of atopy and the relationship of atopy to airway hyper-responsiveness. Another interesting genetic influence on childhood asthma appears to be the sex of the child. Boys are twice as likely to develop asthma in childhood than girls, although this ratio is equal by adolescence. By adult life, females have more asthma than males. A number of differences exist between boys and girls in terms of airway growth and maturation during childhood. Relatively smaller and more responsive airways in males during childhood might account for the observed differences in asthma rates in boys and girls.

2    Environmental factors

(a) *Viral infections*
As mentioned previously, viral infections such as the common cold are the most important trigger factors in childhood asthma. There is also some evidence to suggest that viral infections may cause a transient increase in airway hyper-responsiveness, even in people without asthma, probably by increasing airway inflammation. The relationship between viral infections and the development of asthma is obscured by the possibility that the airways may have been abnormal before the infection, thus causing the child to wheeze. In other words, rather than inducing the asthmatic state, viral-induced wheezing may simply reflect an already sensitive airway. There is also evidence to suggest that airway size may be important in determining whether wheezing occurs in response to a viral infection. This could explain why some children appear to lose their tendency to wheeze as they grow, while those with persistent symptoms may be the ones with hyper-responsive airways. Some of these questions may be answered by studies currently looking at the development of asthma and airway hyper-responsiveness in early infancy.

(b) *Allergens*

The increased association of atopy with more severe and persistent forms of asthma would suggest that allergic factors are important in the development of airway hyper-responsiveness.

Early exposure to food allergens does not appear to be important in the development of asthma. A number of studies have demonstrated that breast feeding and early avoidance of the common foods known to cause allergic reactions, will reduce the rate of eczema and immediate food allergic reactions in infants with a family history of atopy. However, there is no convincing evidence that the rate of asthma or allergic nasal problems is reduced by this dietary manipulation. This provides further evidence that food allergy is not an important cause of asthma.

In contrast airborne allergens do appear to be important in the development and maintenance of airway hyper-responsiveness. While these allergens appear to be less important as triggers of wheezing in childhood, there is good evidence that allergen exposure can increase airway hyper-responsiveness in patients known to be allergic to that particular allergen. This appears to be due to the development of inflammatory changes in the airway as part of the allergic reaction. These mechanisms are only likely to be important in people who have atopy, and do not explain the development of airway hyper-responsiveness in all situations. However, recent evidence would suggest that early exposure to airborne allergens may be critical for the development of the allergic response, which in turn is important for the development of asthma. Further understanding of the development of these IgE responses to inhaled allergens is likely to be very important in any attempt at trying to prevent the development of asthma.

(c) *Smoking*

There is increasing evidence that maternal smoking may be one of the most important influences on the development of airway hyper-responsiveness and asthma. In utero exposure to cigarette smoke has been shown to increase IgE production in some studies. Additionally, infants born to mothers who smoke are more likely to have hyper-responsive airways soon after birth, irrespective of a family history of asthma. The exact mechanism for these findings is still unclear, but one factor may be an effect on growth of the lung, particularly the airways. In addition, passive smoking in infancy has also been shown to increase the risk of developing both atopy and airway hyper-responsiveness. The demonstration that cigarette smoke can influence the development of asthma so early in life, has emphasised the importance of considering exposures to other factors during pregnancy and early infancy as possible contributors to asthma.

(d) *Other factors*

Other trigger factors such as exercise, food additives and emotional stress do not appear to be important in inducing or maintaining airway hyper-responsiveness. While outdoor air pollution is often stated to be the cause of the apparent increase in asthma in recent years, there is currently little definite evidence to suggest that it is a major contributing factor.

---

## SUMMARY: WHAT IS ASTHMA?

- Asthma literally means 'difficulty in breathing'.
- The symptoms of asthma arise because of airway narrowing related to airway muscle contraction, swelling of the airway wall and mucus secretion.
- The airways of the asthmatic are more sensitive, which in turn is thought to reflect the state of persistent inflammation apparent in the airway of the asthmatic subject.
- Certain trigger factors can provoke airway narrowing in these sensitive airways: viral infections are the most important in childhood.
- The development of the asthmatic tendency is related to a number of factors, including inherited and environmental influences and airway size.
- Exposure to airborne allergens and maternal smoking have been identified as important early factors determining the development of asthma in childhood.

# 3

# ASTHMA THROUGH THE AGES

## INTRODUCTION

### Prevalence

Asthma is the commonest cause of recurrent episodes of cough and wheeze in childhood. The estimated prevalence of asthma will vary from country to country and also according to the definition used. However, Australia and New Zealand appear to have the highest prevalence of asthma in the world. Current estimates indicate that asthma symptoms occur in between 25 and 30 per cent of children at some time during childhood, yet asthma is diagnosed in only about half of these children. Although the prevalence of asthma appears to have increased over the last 20 years, it is difficult to determine whether this is simply a reflection of more accurate diagnosis. Thus many children previously labelled as having 'bronchitis' are now more correctly being recognised as suffering from asthma. There remains considerable debate, therefore, as to whether there has been a real increase in asthma prevalence, although some recent evidence does suggest that even allowing for improved recognition, there has been an increase in asthmatic symptoms in childhood. The reasons for such an increase, if real, remain to be determined.

### Severity

While asthma is a very common childhood complaint, the majority of children have relatively mild disease. Asthma can be classified in childhood as:
- (a) episodic (intermittent episodes of cough and wheeze) or
- (b) persistent (troublesome symptoms present on most days).

Episodic asthma can be further arbitrarily subdivided according to severity into infrequent or frequent episodic asthma. Episodic asthma accounts for 95 per cent of children with asthma, with two-thirds having infrequent and one-third having frequent episodes. Thus only five per cent of children with asthma would be classified as having persistent asthma and less than one per cent would be considered as having very severe asthma. This classification is useful when considering the assessment of children with asthma and will be discussed in more detail in Chapter 4.

## Age of onset

While asthma can develop at any age, around 50 per cent of children develop their asthma in the first three years and about 80 per cent will have developed symptoms by seven years of age. There is a male predominance of children suffering from asthma, with boys also tending to have more severe forms of asthma. Thus, asthma occurs about twice as commonly in boys than girls but while infrequent asthma occurs equally in boys and girls, persistent asthma is four times more common in boys. This effect is lost by puberty with approximately equal numbers of males and females developing asthma at this age, and by adult life females tend to develop asthma more commonly.

The remainder of this chapter will highlight unique features of asthma during different ages from infancy to adolescence and expand on some of the issues raised in Chapter 1.

## THE WHEEZY BABY

### 'Infantile Asthma'

Wheezing is a common symptom in the first year of life, although it is often difficult to make a definite diagnosis in this age group. This is due to the fact that wheezing in infancy appears to be related more to airway size than to airway hyper-responsiveness. Thus in many infants, a tendency to wheeze appears to be restricted to the first year or so of life, and then settles as the airway grows. While the term 'infantile asthma' is often used to describe wheezing infants, it is clear that many do not have the typical features of asthma. In particular these infants are often poorly responsive to the usual anti-asthma medications (both bronchodilators and preventive treatments). Often they are not particularly distressed by their wheezing, continuing to eat, sleep, grow and develop normally while 'wheezing' and 'rattling' their way through their first years of life. These infants have often been described as 'fat happy wheezers' and they tend to worry their parents and attending physician more than they distress themselves.

While this form of wheezing is often attributed to cow's milk allergy, there is little evidence to implicate cow's milk as the cause of wheezing in the majority of these infants. While a trial of anti-asthma treatment may be indicated in some of these infants, particularly during colds, their response to treatment is often disappointing, as mentioned previously. Therefore, a decision to continue treatment should be based on their response to initial

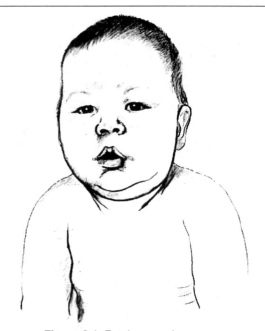

**Figure 3.1**: Fat, happy wheezer

therapy as well as their degree of distress, in order to ensure that treatment is not continued unnecessarily.

In the long term, most infants with typical 'infantile asthma' appear to have a favourable outcome. About half of these infants outgrow their tendency to wheeze about the age of 12 or 18 months, and are not subsequently troubled by cough or wheeze. The other half develop more typical symptoms of asthma, particularly with colds. They usually follow the episodic pattern, often the infrequent variety, and between 12 and 18 months of age will start to respond to asthma medications.

## Severe infantile asthma

There does appear to be a small subgroup of infants who present with more typical asthma symptoms in the first year of life. These infants have recurrent episodes of wheezing, often associated with significant difficulty in breathing. They may require hospitalisation for treatment and interestingly, appear to be more responsive to anti-asthma treatment, although often require regular preventive treatment to obtain good control of their asthma. These infants usually have a strong family history of asthma or other allergic diseases and will often have eczema, persistent nasal symptoms or food allergic reactions associated with their tendency to wheeze. These infants are more likely to follow a pattern of persistent asthma throughout childhood, although some may again revert to a predominantly episodic pattern after the first year of life.

## Investigations

While these two patterns of wheezing account for the majority of infants presenting with recurrent or persistent wheezing, there are a number of other disorders which may need to be considered. The need for further investigation will be determined by your doctor according to your infant's progress. Often a simple investigation such as a chest X-ray can be useful to decide whether further tests are warranted.

## Bronchiolitis and asthma

The other common cause of an acute episode of wheezing in infants under 12 months of age is infection with respiratory syncytial virus (RSV). This produces an illness termed viral bronchiolitis which is characterised initially by symptoms of a common cold, but in which cough, wheeze and breathing difficulty eventually develop. This usually occurs as a winter epidemic and some infants require hospitalisation for observation and treatment. There remains considerable debate about the relationship between infection with RSV and the development of asthma. While hospital-based studies have suggested that RSV infection is associated with an increased likelihood of developing asthma, this may simply reflect a predisposition to develop wheezing rather than a consequence of infection. Thus the need for hospitalisation with RSV might be the first indication of asthma in these infants. Long-term studies of infants followed from birth, which are currently being performed, may help to resolve this issue.

## THE PRE-SCHOOL CHILD

### Pattern of asthma

This age group represents the peak prevalence of asthma during childhood. Episodic asthma predominates and episodes are usually associated with viral infections such as the common cold. An average child will have six to eight respiratory infections a year in the first five to six years of life, and any tendency to wheeze will complicate these infections. A common pattern for the asthmatic child in this age group, if not appropriately treated, is to cough and wheeze through most of winter, a time when respiratory viruses are most prevalent. The frequency of wheezing episodes can vary significantly from child to child, and is probably the reflection of both the underlying sensitivity of the airway and the nature of the virus. Some children may only have two or three wheezing episodes in their lifetime while others will wheeze with each of their respiratory infections. These children with very frequent

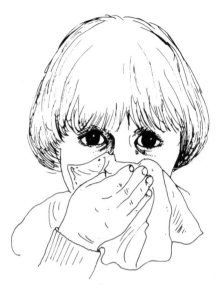

**Figure 3.2**: Pre-school child with cold

episodes of wheezing may take much longer to recover from their episodes, often being left with a cough at night or induced by exercise for several weeks. Others have more troublesome wheezing between these more acute episodes and would be classified as having persistent asthma. The frequency of episodes of wheezing and presence of symptoms between episodes are useful measures when assessing severity of asthma.

## Recurrent cough

Another common presentation of asthma in the pre-school years is with cough as the predominant and sometimes the only symptom. When the cough is mainly episodic, associated with colds, it can be difficult to distinguish asthma as the cause of the cough from viral bronchitis, that is, inflammation of the airway related to infection with the virus. Some clues to the diagnosis of asthma include the dry irritating nature of the cough, the persistence of cough between infections or associated wheezing. Although the cough tends to be worse at night, this is not necessarily a distinguishing feature from viral bronchitis. However associated exercise-related symptoms might be more suggestive of asthma. The presence of other allergic problems such as eczema or hay fever in the child or a family history of asthma or other allergic disease, would also point to asthma as being the cause of the cough. Investigations are usually not all that helpful in this age group as children are generally too young to perform reliable measurements of lung function.

Therefore, it is often left to a trial of asthma medication to confirm any suspicion of asthma. Interestingly, bronchodilators appear to be less effective in children with cough as the predominant symptom, suggesting that inflammatory pathology such as mucus production and swelling of the airway wall are more important than muscle constriction. Thus preventive medication is often needed to control the cough, particularly when symptoms are frequent.

## Hyper-secretory asthma

Another variant of asthma which is important to recognise is so-called 'hyper-secretory asthma'. As the name implies, increased mucus secretion is the predominant change. Cough is therefore the principal symptom, and often the cough can sound very 'rattly' because of the mucus present in the airways. More important, this mucus in the airways can block off the air reaching the air sacs and therefore cause collapse of small areas of the lung. This is often interpreted on chest X-ray as infection of the air sacs (pneumonia) rather than due to mucus plugging the airways. These children may then be labelled as having 'recurrent pneumonia', whereas in fact, asthma is the cause of their problem. Again, use of appropriate anti-asthma medication will usually help to confirm the diagnosis and at the same time provide relief from symptoms.

## Other causes of cough and wheeze

While asthma is again the most common cause of recurrent episodes of cough and wheeze in this age group, other causes may need to be considered in your child if there are atypical features or if response to anti-asthma treatment is poor. Of particular importance is the inhalation of foreign materials into the airways. Toddlers often put things in their mouths and from there they can easily be inhaled. Onset of symptoms after a 'choking' episode, persistence of symptoms despite adequate treatment or persistent chest X-ray abnormalities, should raise the possibility of an inhaled foreign body (*see* Figure 3.3).

## THE SCHOOL-AGE CHILD

## Pattern of asthma

During the school-age years, many children with episodic asthma, particularly those with infrequent episodes, cease wheezing. Therefore, the prevalence of current asthma (asthma in the past 12 months) falls gradually from the time of school entry to the teenage years. However, those with continuing asthma symptoms tend to be those at the more severe end of the asthma spectrum. While the frequency of acute episodes generally lessens in this age group, associated with the reduced rate of viral respiratory infections,

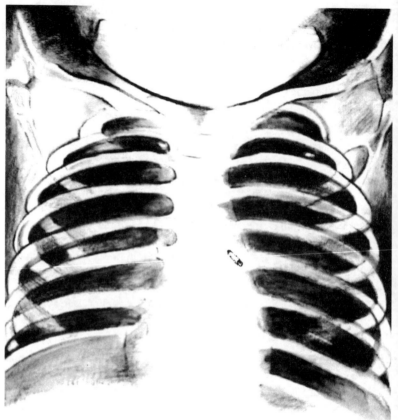

**Figure 3.3**: Foreign body X-ray demonstrating a safety pin in the bronchus

many of these children will have persistent low-grade symptoms which can often be overlooked. Therefore, it is important that they continue to be carefully monitored and receive appropriate preventive therapy when indicated.

## Exercise-induced asthma

Exercise-induced asthma becomes an increasingly important problem for the school-age child, and may be the presenting feature of asthma in this age group. As children participate in more competitive sporting endeavours, their level of exercise increases and thus the likelihood of provoking exercise-induced wheezing increases. It is important to ensure that the asthmatic child is not restricted in his or her ability to exercise or compete with peers. Therefore, encouraging activity, with the use of appropriate pre-exercise treatment should be high on the list of priorities for the school-age child with asthma.

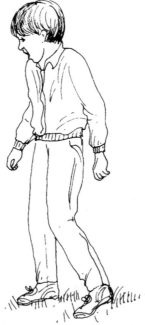

**Figure 3.4**: Child with exercise-induced asthma

## Coping with asthma at school

Parents often have concern about how their child will cope with an episode of asthma at school. This can be addressed at several levels. It is important for parents to inform the school of their child's asthma and to indicate to the teacher any treatment required regularly, or what to do in the event of an attack.

School staff are being encouraged to become more aware of asthma and also to encourage students with asthma to seek education about their condition. In addition, it has been suggested that students be allowed to carry their medications on their persons and that a bronchodilator aerosol be available in the first aid kit. Thus it is likely that teachers will be receptive to your approach regarding your child's asthma.

## Encouraging independence

It is also important for you to encourage your child to understand asthma and its treatment, and to allow him/her to take increasing responsibility for their asthma management as they grow older. Therapy can usually be tailored to interfere minimally with school and school activities. Use of appropriate preventive therapy should reduce the amount of school lost through asthma and *at the same time* allow your child to participate in normal school activities. By fostering your child's interest in understanding and managing their asthma during the primary school years, they should reach their adolescence with the ability to cope with their asthma during the difficult teenage years.

## ADOLESCENCE

### Asthma and the adolescent

Adolescence is a difficult time for the normal child, let alone one needing to face the added burden of a chronic disease. Although the prevalence of asthma in the teenage years is less than that in early childhood, asthma accounts for over 25 per cent of chronic illness in this age group. There is also a relative increase in the number with persistent or frequent episodic asthma, and these children will require regular treatment to keep them well controlled. Normal adolescence is about dealing with the changes of puberty, establishing a healthy body image and gaining independence. Anything that threatens these pursuits may affect the teenagers' ability to cope with these normal adolescent conflicts. Although the majority of children with asthma will progress through the pubertal changes at the normal time, some with severe persistent asthma will have pubertal delay related to their chronic disease. These children will therefore be short during early adolescence but long-term studies have indicated that catch up growth occurs and these children achieve normal stature. This growth delay appears more related to the disease than to its therapy, as aggressive treatment in those with poor control of asthma symptoms often results in catch up growth. The nature and cause of this pubertal delay needs to be explained to the teenager, and reassurance can be given of a normal outcome.

### Coping with a chronic disease

Coping with a chronic disease which requires regular treatment can interfere with the development of both body image and independence. Some teenagers may adopt the 'sick' role, remaining very dependent on their parents to manage their asthma. Many others, preoccupied with being 'normal' deny their disease and become poorly compliant with treatment.

Managing the adolescent with asthma can prove a difficult task for both parent and doctor. The establishment of self-management skills during the later childhood years may be very helpful in allowing teenagers to cope with their asthma, as mentioned earlier. The emphasis should be on their ability to control their disease with appropriate treatment aimed at normalising their lifestyle. Independence should be encouraged, but at the same time support should be offered when needed.

There needs to be a gradual transition from the medical consultation with parents present, to that with the teenager alone, and the age at which this occurs may vary for each individual. Encouraging the adolescent to take responsibility for his or her disease and then, emphasising the positive aspects of controlling the disease, helps to address the issues mentioned previously. At the same time, it is important for the doctor to ensure that the treatment program is realistic and flexible, allowing the teenager some input into discussions about management.

## Adolescent risk-taking

Adolescence is also a time of risk-taking behaviour. This can be manifest in the asthmatic patient in a number of ways. Cessation of medication which may lead to worsening asthma, is an example of risk-taking behaviour which may lead to non-compliance with treatment. Cigarette smoking is another example of such behaviour. There is tremendous pressure on the teenager to experiment and, despite the adverse publicity that cigarette smoking has had recently, the number of smoking teenagers remains high. In a follow-up of asthmatic children at age 21 years, it was noted that 40 per cent smoked. It is to be hoped that the increasing evidence of the harmful effects of both active and passive smoking on the lungs, will help reduce this problem. Clearly asthmatic children need to be encouraged from an early age to *avoid* smoke exposure, and this message needs to be *repeated* during adolescence.

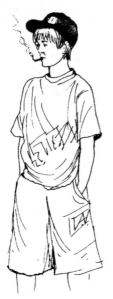

**Figure 3.5**: Adolescent risk-taking

## Emotional factors

Emotional factors may become more prominent in the adolescent with asthma. Anxiety may be manifest by hyper-ventilation episodes which complicate the management of their asthma. Emotional triggers may also exacerbate episodes of acute wheezing related to other triggers. Children with severe persistent asthma appear to be at most risk for associated emotional problems. In some situations, counselling, family assessment and family therapy have proved very helpful in identifying and addressing emotional factors contributing to poor asthma control.

---

### SUMMARY: ASTHMA THROUGH THE AGES

- Asthmatic symptoms occur in 25-30 per cent of children
- Asthma in childhood may be divided into episodic (in 95 per cent of cases) and persistent (in five per cent of cases).
- Around 50 per cent of children develop their asthma in the first three years of life and 80 per cent by seven years of age.
- Boys develop asthma in childhood about twice as often as girls, and also tend to have more severe asthma.
- Wheezing in infancy is common and may not necessarily indicate asthma.
- Episodic asthma predominates in the pre-school child and is usually related to viral infections. Cough may be the presenting symptom.
- Exercise-induced asthma is an important problem for the school-age child. Adjusting to school may also be an important issue.
- The adolescent with asthma must learn to cope with a chronic disease during normal adolescent development. Emphasis should be on allowing self-management and independence.

# 4

# ASSESSING SEVERITY

## INTRODUCTION

In order to decide what treatment will be appropriate for a child with asthma, it is useful to categorise the severity of the asthma. For simplicity, asthma in childhood can be classified as:

(a)   Mild: Infrequent episodic asthma (70 per cent)
(b)   Moderate: Frequent episodic asthma (25 per cent)
(c)   Severe: Persistent asthma (5 per cent)

While this is clearly an arbitrary means of classification, it does provide a useful basis for assessing severity and prescribing treatment as will be discussed in Chapter 8. It should also be noted that children may change from one group to the other, either worsening because of an increase in airway hyper-responsiveness or improving because of treatment or time. Thus reassessment should be performed at regular intervals and treatment varied according to the progress of the child's asthma.

Assessing the severity of a child's asthma should be a joint exercise for the parent, with the involvement of the older child or adolescent, and the doctor. Diary card recordings of the frequency of symptoms and the need for medication as well as home peak flow monitoring in the older child provides very important information for the doctor to categorise your child's asthma. Assessment of asthma severity is based on three main factors:

1   Clinical history
2   Physical examination
3   Lung function testing

The use and limitations of these assessments will be discussed in this chapter and a summary appears in Table 4.1.

## CLINICAL HISTORY

A carefully taken history of the frequency and nature of asthma symptoms forms the basis of the assessment and classification of asthma severity. This history will have to be obtained from the parents of the younger child, which

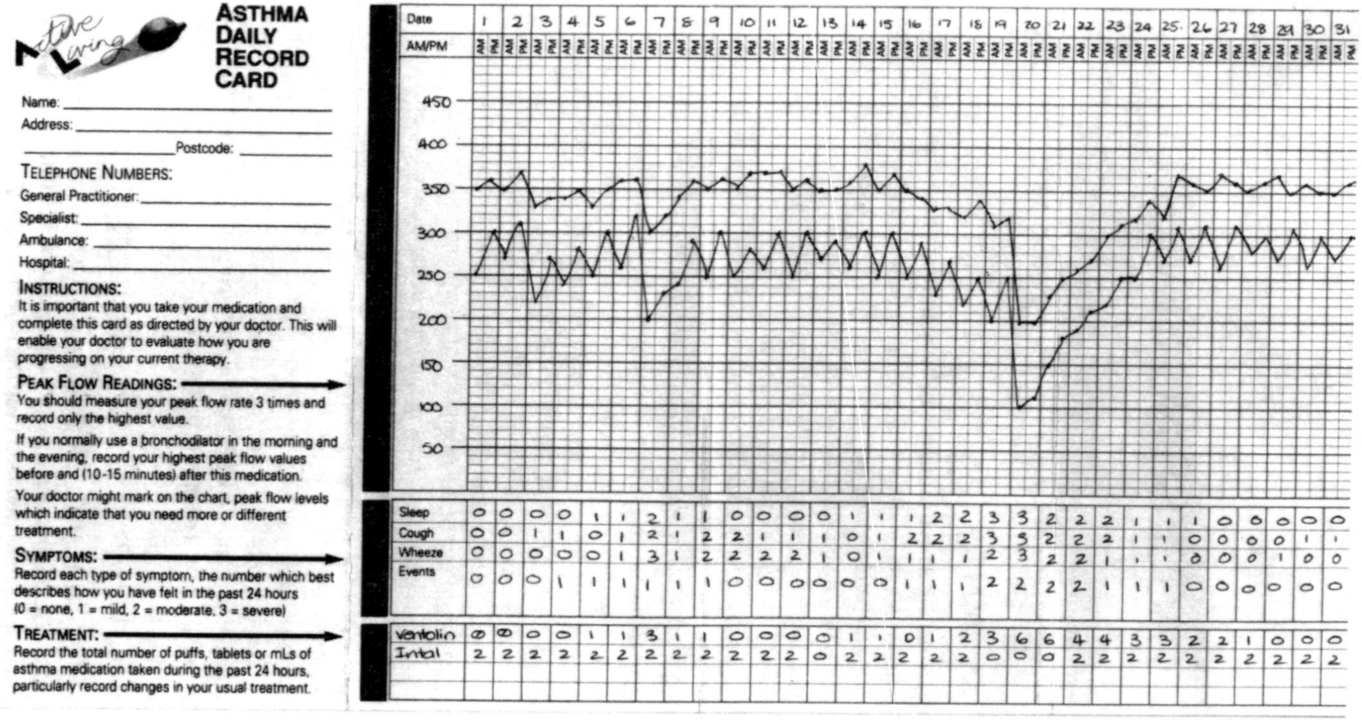
Active Living
ASTHMA DAILY RECORD CARD
Name:
Address:
Postcode:
TELEPHONE NUMBERS:
General Practitioner:
Specialist:
Ambulance:
Hospital:
INSTRUCTIONS:
It is important that you take your medication and complete this card as directed by your doctor. This will enable your doctor to evaluate how you are progressing on your current therapy.
PEAK FLOW READINGS:
You should measure your peak flow rate 3 times and record only the highest value.
If you normally use a bronchodilator in the morning and the evening, record your highest peak flow values before and (10-15 minutes) after this medication.
Your doctor might mark on the chart, peak flow levels which indicate that you need more or different treatment.
SYMPTOMS:
Record each type of symptom, the number which best describes how you have felt in the past 24 hours (0 = none, 1 = mild, 2 = moderate, 3 = severe)
TREATMENT:
Record the total number of puffs, tablets or mLs of asthma medication taken during the past 24 hours, particularly record changes in your usual treatment.
Date
AM/PM
450
400
350
300
250
200
150
100
50
Sleep
Cough
Wheeze
Events
Ventolin
Intal

Figure 4.1: Diary card

**Table 4.1:** Severity of asthma

| | Mild (Infrequent episodic) | Moderate (Frequent episodic) | Severe (Persistent) |
|---|---|---|---|
| **Clinical history** | | | |
| Frequency of acute episodes (per year) | <6 | 6–12 | >12 |
| Interval symptoms | Absent | Mild | Moderate-Severe |
| Lifestyle disruption | Absent | Mild | Moderate-Severe |
| Bronchodilator usage (average per week) | <2–3 | >2–3 | Daily |
| **Physical Examination** (between episodes) | Normal | Normal | Abnormal |
| **Spirometry** (between episodes) | Normal | Normal | Abnormal |
| **PEFR Variability** | <30% | 30–50% | >50% |

introduces the difficulty of having to rely on a third party, which is never as good as a history obtained directly from the patient. There is often a tendency to underestimate the frequency and severity of asthma symptoms, particularly in the child with persistent asthma. In this situation, the child and the family often learn to 'live with their asthma' that is, their ability to recognise symptoms is reduced because they constantly have some degree of airway narrowing and have learned to adapt. Therefore, specific questions, as outlined below: diary card monitoring and lung function testing (if the child is old enough to perform this reliably) can help in the estimation of severity.

The following questions are very helpful in classifying childhood asthma into the different categories of asthma severity:

1    How frequently do attacks of asthma occur?
     This is most useful in those children with episodic asthma as children with persistent asthma may not recognise discrete attacks. If episodes occur every six to eight weeks, or more frequently then the child has frequent episodic asthma and is considered to be at least moderate in severity. Children with mild or infrequent episodic asthma will have a variable frequency from two or three episodes in a life-time to three or four episodes a year.

2    How severe are the attacks?
     The nature and duration of the attacks and the nature and response to treatment are important factors in assessing the severity of an acute episode of asthma. The presence of collapse or fainting, blueness of the

lips (cyanosis) or the need for hospitalisation (other than with the first episode) classify the episode as severe.

3    Does the child have symptoms between attacks?

The presence of night-time cough, early morning cough or wheeze or exercise-induced cough or wheeze which persist between episodes of asthma are signs of more severe asthma.

Children with moderate (frequent episodic) asthma may have some degree of low-grade symptoms, particularly following an acute episode. This probably relates to a transient increase in airway hyper-responsiveness following the acute episode, which is usually triggered by a viral infection. A usual pattern is for these children to have a persistent cough through the winter months but to be free of symptoms through summer.

Children with severe (persistent) asthma will have more troublesome symptoms on a daily basis and apparently unrelated to acute episodes. They will often wake at night requiring their bronchodilator medication and on rising in the morning may feel 'tight' in the chest and again need their medication. They will also tend to be wheezy during the day, particularly with exercise, and are often significantly restricted in their exercise tolerance. The children will often react to a wide variety of trigger factors. This tendency to have widely varying degrees of airway narrowing is often termed 'labile asthma'.

4    Is the child's lifestyle affected by his or her asthma?

(a) Sleep disturbance

Night-time symptoms are common in asthma, because airway hyper-responsiveness tends to be worse in the early morning hours, the child often waking at two or three in the morning.

Sleep disturbance is common during an acute episode of wheezing but persistent sleep disturbance between episodes is a sign of more severe asthma which requires intensification of treatment.

(b) Exercise tolerance

Exercise-induced wheezing is a good index of asthma severity, as it closely reflects the degree of airway hyper-responsiveness. Therefore, the degree to which a child's ability to exercise is restricted, is a good index of asthma severity.

When assessing exercise tolerance, it is important also to assess what exercise the child is actually doing. Many children with persistent asthma simply don't exercise because they know it will provoke their asthma. They will not complain of exercise intolerance or exercise-induced wheezing. Thus it is important to know how much exercise the child with asthma can actually do.

(c) School absence

The amount of time lost from school, or pre-school, due to asthma is also a good index of severity. Both the reason for the absence and the frequency of such absences will help to differentiate those with episodic asthma from those with more persistent forms of asthma.

(d) Hospitalisation

The frequency and duration of hospitalisation also provides a good index of asthma severity. As mentioned previously, the need for hospitalisation for an acute episode immediately suggests that the episode was of moderate severity. It should therefore call for a re-assessment of the child's asthma and may well prompt a change in treatment.

Children who require repeated admissions to hospital either for acute episodes or for more chronic symptoms should be classified as having more severe asthma than children with a similar symptom pattern who have never been hospitalised.

5    How frequently are bronchodilators needed to treat symptoms of cough and/or wheeze?

As bronchodilator inhalers (Ventolin, Respolin, Bricanyl or Berotec) are usually used as first-line treatment for symptomatic relief, the frequency with which they are used will reflect asthma severity. It is also important to make an assessment of bronchodilator usage, as the current aim of treatment is to limit the need for bronchodilator medication by using appropriate preventive medication.

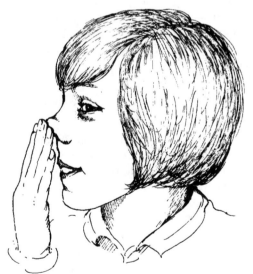

**Figure 4.2**: Nasal crease and 'allergic shiner'

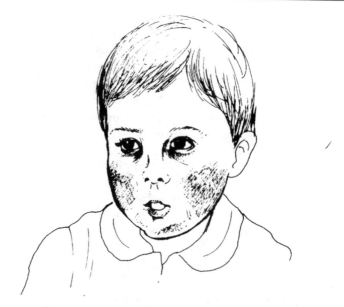

**Figure 4.3**: Child with atopic dermatitis/eczema

It is often difficult for the child or parent to recall how many times a day the bronchodilator puffer has been used. This can be recorded as part of a diary card assessment, on a daily basis, to overcome this problem. In addition, the need to repurchase a bronchodilator puffer at frequent intervals should signal asthma which is poorly controlled. For example, a child who uses a Ventolin puffer in one week, is needing two puffs on average 14 times a day. This would be an indication to revise the preventive treatment.

## PHYSICAL EXAMINATION

Assuming that the child is between acute episodes of wheezing, children with episodic asthma should have an essentially normal physical examination.

The presence of wheezing between episodes (either audible or with a stethoscope) should immediately alert the doctor to the possibility of persistent asthma. In children with 'labile' asthma, wheezing may be provoked by coughing or running. The presence of a deformity of the chest wall (pigeon or barrel chest) or of the lower end of the rib cage (Harrison's sulci) is also suggestive of chronic under-treated asthma. In addition, the growth pattern of the child may also reflect severe asthma, as fall off in growth (initially weight then height) may be a sign of increasing asthma severity. Children with more severe disease will often have evidence of other allergic problems, for example, chronic flexural eczema or nasal allergy with blocked nose; 'allergic shiners' (black rings under the eyes) and a crease across the nose from constant rubbing of the 'itchy' nose (transverse nasal crease).

Physical examination evidence of persistent asthma in a child who is historically well at the time of examination, should signal the possibility that the clinical history of the child's asthma severity has been underestimated. In this situation, diary card recordings and monitoring of lung function may be helpful in confirming this suspicion.

## LUNG FUNCTION

The measurement of lung function provides an objective assessment of the degree of airway narrowing and the response of this narrowing to broncho-dilator medication.

Ideally, lung function should be measured at some time in all children with asthma. However, from a practical viewpoint, children under the age of five years will not be able to perform simple lung function tests reliably. There-fore lung function assessment will usually be limited to children of five years and over, while clinical history and physical examination will remain the main means of assessment in children under five years of age.

The principle behind measuring lung function in asthma is that airway narrowing will reduce the rate at which air flows while breathing out. This reduction in the rate that air leaves the lung will increase the time it takes to empty the lung fully. However, apart from severe forms of asthma, when air can be trapped in the lung, the total amount of air that the asthmatic child can exhale will be normal.

Lung function in asthmatic children can be measured in two different ways:

1   Spirometry
    Spirometry is a procedure which allows measurement of airflow at different lung volumes, from a maximum breath in, to a maximum breath out. As reduction in airflow in asthma is often demonstrated only at low lung volumes it is a sensitive measure of airway narrowing.
    This procedure is usually performed in a laboratory or doctor's office as the equipment required is currently not easily portable.
    Baseline spirometry is performed when the child is 'well'. In children with episodic asthma who would be expected to have no evidence of airway narrowing between attacks, spirometry should be normal. In contrast, children with persistent asthma are likely to have persisting evidence of airway narrowing between attacks, reflected by reduced air-flow rates, with an improvement after bronchodilator medication. To ensure that bronchodilator medication does not mask the presence of

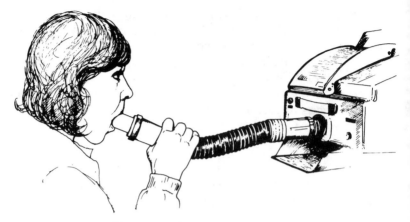

**Figure 4.4**: Child using a spirometer

airway narrowing, this is usually withheld for a period of time before testing.

Spirometry can also be useful for the assessment of the severity of an acute episode of wheezing. However, many children are too distressed to perform the required manoeuvre reliably, and this must be taken into account when interpreting the results.

For the measurement of spirometry, the child is asked to take a maximal breath in and blow out as hard and fast as possible – like blowing out candles on a birthday cake. The ability to perform this manoeuvre will obviously affect the interpretation of the results and this is particularly important in young children or those with an acute episode of wheezing. An analysis of the child's technique and the results produced will usually differentiate between abnormal results which are real or artefactual.

Airflow rates are usually calculated as the best of two or three attempts and then expressed as a percentage of normal predicted values. An analysis of the results allows an estimation of the degree of airway narrowing and its reversibility with bronchodilator medication. Serial measurements may be useful in documenting effects of changes in treatment.

2    Home peak flow monitoring

Peak expiratory flow rate (PEFR) measures the airflow at the maximum lung volume, that is, when the child starts to breathe out after a maximal breathe in. It is a less-sensitive (though much simpler) measurement of airway narrowing than spirometry but is very dependent on effort.

While spirometry is a more sensitive measurement of airway narrowing than PEFR, at present its expense and lack of portability makes it

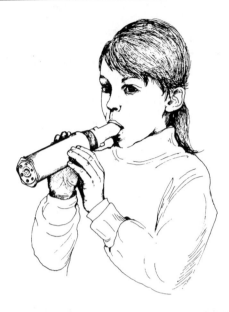

**Figure 4.5**: Using the peak expiratory flow meter (PEFR)

difficult to use for home monitoring. In addition, normal spirometric results on a single occasion do not exclude the possibility that a child with asthma may have varying degrees of airway narrowing at different times on the same day. Therefore home PEFR monitoring should be seen as supplementary to spirometry in the assessment of asthma severity.[1]

The measurement of PEFR involves the child taking a deep breath in and blowing out maximally. This measures the flow rate only at the beginning of expiration. PEFR is a relatively insensitive measurement of airway narrowing and does not become abnormal till airway narrowing is moderate to severe. However, the variability in measurements of PEFR, both at different times during the day and before and after bronchodilator medication, has been shown to reflect airway hyper-responsiveness and therefore, asthma severity to some degree. PEFR variability is usually expressed as:

$$\frac{\text{Highest PEFR} - \text{Lowest PEFR} \times 100 \text{ per cent}}{\text{Highest PEFR (or mean PEFR)}}$$

---

1 PEFR monitors are available through pharmacies, hospitals and Asthma Foundations and generally cost between $20 to $30. The need for PEFR monitoring in your child should be discussed with your doctor, as in many children with asthma, it will be unnecessary.

44

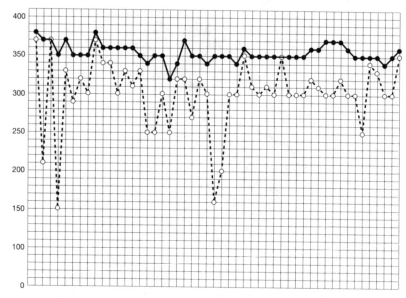

**Figure 4.6**: PEFR variability (after preventive treatment)

and an estimation of the mean PEFR variability over a period of time can be used as a measure of severity. In children, PEFR variability up to 20 per cent is generally considered within the normal range; 20 to 30 per cent indicates mild asthma; 30 to 50 per cent moderate asthma and greater than 50 per cent severe asthma.

While PEFR measurements do provide a reliable indicator of asthma severity, there are some limitations in childhood:

(a) Age

In general, children under five years will not perform a reliable PEFR and results must be interpreted *carefully* in this age group.

(b) Effort dependence

The measurement of PEFR depends to a large extent on the effort the child puts into this manoeuvre. Thus, in young children and children with an acute episode of wheezing, a low PEFR may reflect poor *effort* rather than severe airway narrowing. Cough may also interfere with the PEFR manoeuvre.

(c) Episodic nature of asthma

The large majority of children who have episodic asthma are likely to have normal lung function between episodes. While establishing a normal baseline reading in these children may be useful to confirm the episodic nature of their disease, regular PEFR monitoring is usually not necessary.

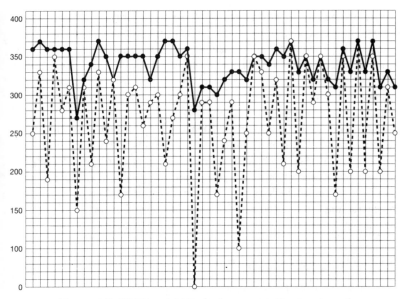

**Figure 4.6**: PEFR variability (before preventive treatment)

Children with asthma who benefit most from PEFR monitoring are therefore older children, with more persistent asthma, or those in whom there is difficulty with, or doubts about, the reliability of the clinical history of asthma symptoms. In these situations, regular monitoring over a period of four to six weeks will establish a baseline and, with the help of diary card monitoring of symptoms, may indicate the need for additional treatment. Depending on these initial results, PEFR monitoring may be additionally needed till control is achieved – at times of acute or increasing symptoms – or if changes in treatment are contemplated.

The further development of home spirometers currently under evaluation, should allow a decision as to whether these more sensitive measures of airway narrowing add any further information to our ability to assess the severity of asthma, based on lung function measurements.

## ASSESSING THE ACUTE EPISODE

Assessing the severity of an acute episode is important as it will dictate the treatment that the child will require. Simple observational measures, such as how fast the child is breathing, how distressed the child is with breathing and what is the level of activity, are useful in the assessment. If the child has had repeated episodes, parents can often compare the severity with previous episodes and therefore, predict the outcome and what might be appropriate treatment. The child may also be able to indicate his or her perception of the severity of the current episode compared with previous episodes.

Perhaps the most useful indicator of asthma severity is the response to bronchodilator medication. If the child's symptoms are relieved with bronchodilator and that relief is maintained for at least four hours, then one could consider that the episode was under reasonable control. Poor response to bronchodilator or short duration of effect, should signal the need for additional therapy according to an Action Plan, which will be discussed in more detail in Chapter 9.

In addition to the clinical assessment, children who are old enough to perform reliable PEFR measurements, can use this additional information to help make decisions about treatment. Once a baseline period of PEFR measurements has been obtained, your doctor will be able to incorporate critical PEFR readings which require additional treatment into the Action Plan. In general, the PEFR response to bronchodilator medication will determine the changes in treatment which are needed during the acute episode.

---

SUMMARY: ASSESSING SEVERITY

- Childhood asthma may be arbitrarily divided into three groups of severity:
  1 Mild: Infrequent episodic asthma
  2 Moderate: Frequent episodic asthma
  3 Severe: Persistent asthma
- Classification of asthma severity is based on:
  1 Clinical history
  2 Physical examination
  3 Lung function testing
- The best historical predictors of asthma severity are: frequency and severity of episodes; presence of symptoms between episodes; lifestyle disruption and the need for bronchodilator medication.
- Physical findings which suggest severe persistent asthma include: poor growth; chest wall deformity and wheezing when 'well'.
- Lung function testing is an important objective measurement of asthma severity in children old enough to perform it reliably. Both spirometry and home PEFR monitoring have a role in this assessment.
- Assessing the severity of an acute episode of wheezing must take into account the child's appearance and response to bronchodilator medication, aided in the older child by measurement of lung function.

# 5

# TRIGGERS – AVOIDABLE OR NOT?

## INTRODUCTION

The ideal way of treating asthma would be to avoid or modify those factors which induce airway hyper-responsiveness or which trigger the airways to narrow. However, in reality, many of these factors are difficult to avoid. Therefore, the need to consider applying avoidance measures will vary with the severity of asthma. Children with persistent asthma are likely to benefit more from environmental manipulation than those with infrequent episodic asthma.

The ease of avoidance or modification also needs to be taken into account. Thus the use of measures to prevent exercise-induced wheezing, when this is problem, should be applied universally. In contrast, the need to apply stringent house dust mite avoidance measures should be carefully assessed, because of the difficulties and expense of achieving effective reduction. Moreover, the allergic status of the child to foods and airborne allergens should be established *before* attempting to exclude these allergens from the environment.

It is therefore important that the need for avoidance measures in your child is discussed with your doctor, so that appropriate and feasible measures are applied.

## EXERCISE

As mentioned previously, exercise-induced wheezing or breathlessness is a common symptom in childhood asthma and also reflects, to some degree, the severity of the child's asthma. One of the aims of asthma treatment is to allow the child to perform exercise normally with his or her peers, so avoiding exercise is not the practical answer to preventing exercise-induced wheezing. Modification of the tendency to wheeze with exercise is readily achievable and is a better solution than treating the wheeze once it has arisen. Most important, the ability to exercise without wheeze demonstrates to the child, his or her ability to compete successfully with peers, despite having asthma.

Prevention of exercise-induced wheezing may be achieved in two main ways, which can be used to complement each other.

**1** Pre-treatment immediately before exercise

(a) *Medication*

The use of an inhaled Beta agonist bronchodilator medication (Ventolin, Respolin, Bricanyl, Berotec) immediately before exercise has been shown to prevent the airway narrowing associated with exercise in about 90 per cent of patients. The duration of the protective effective is generally less than two hours, so repeated doses may be needed if duration of exercise is prolonged. If the child develops symptoms of wheezing during prolonged exercise, it is advisable that the child receive an additional dose of bronchodilator medication and rest till the symptoms have subsided.

Another medication which has been shown to be effective in preventing exercise-induced wheezing is sodium cromoglycate (Intal). This has been shown to prevent both the immediate response to exercise and also the late response (six to eight hours after exercise) which may occur in up to 30 per cent of children with severe exercise-

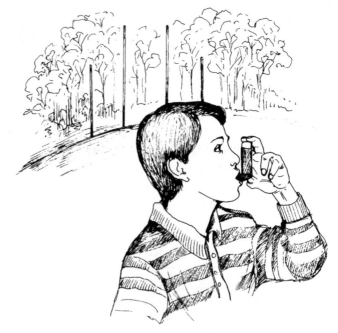

**Figure 5.1**: Using a puffer before sport

induced asthma. As this medication has no major bronchodilator effect, additional bronchodilator medication may be needed if symptoms of airway narrowing occur. In children with troublesome exercise-induced wheezing, a combination of a Beta agonist bronchodilator and sodium cromoglycate can be used, as there does appear to be some additive benefit. However, the need for this level of pre-treatment should also signal the need for re-assessment of regular preventive therapy.

(b) *Warm-up sprints*

The tendency to wheeze after exercise has also been shown to be reduced by performing a series of 30-second sprints at two minute intervals in the 30 minute period before exercise. These warm-up exercises can be used as an alternative, or in addition to, medication, depending on how much protection is achieved with their use.

2    Regular preventive therapy

(a) *Medication*

As the severity of exercise-induced asthma is usually a good index of asthma severity, the use of regular preventive medication, such as sodium cromoglycate or inhaled corticosteroid medications, can be used as a means of reducing the tendency for airway narrowing to occur after exercise. This concept of regular medication to reduce the tendency of airways to narrow, will be addressed in more detail in subsequent chapters.

(b) *Exercise training*

While physical fitness has not been shown to alter the natural history of asthma, it does have some positive benefits for the asthmatic child. Physical fitness does allow the child to undertake greater degrees of exercise, without developing exercise-induced asthma. In addition, physical fitness allows the child to cope better with acute airway narrowing due to other triggers.

Many patients with asthma have been able to achieve in sport at the highest level by learning ways to modify their tendency to wheeze with exercise. There is *no* reason why the child with asthma cannot aspire to similar sporting success.

## AIR POLLUTION

1    Outdoor air pollution

As mentioned previously, the role of outdoor air pollution in provoking asthma has generally been over-emphasised and levels of pollutants in most cities in Australia are well below those at which effects on the respiratory tract are usually seen. It is, nevertheless, important to ensure that levels of ozone, sulphur dioxide, nitrogen dioxide and other particulate matter remain at acceptable levels in our community, as these all have the potential to increase the severity of asthmatic symptoms.

Many parents feel that asthma is more common in certain parts of the country and that moving from these apparent 'high risk' areas may improve their child's asthma. The prevalence of asthma is very similar in the major capital cities of Australia and in both coastal and inland towns, where prevalence has been documented. Thus, in reality, moving house is unlikely to bring an instant cure to the disease, although there is sometimes a 'honeymoon' period where the child appears to improve in the short term, only to redevelop symptoms after some time. Although this apparent improvement may relate to avoidance of some trigger factors not present in the new environment, many triggers, for example, a viral infection, will be common, and some different trigger factors may be unique to the new environment. In most situations, moving from an apparently 'highly polluted' area to one of 'low pollution' will *not* produce a dramatic change in the severity of asthma.

2    Cigarette smoke

Cigarette smoke remains *the* most important indoor air pollutant and cigarette smoke exposure, both active and passive, has been strongly linked with the development of asthma.

It is therefore important that parents of asthmatic children make a positive effort to eliminate cigarette smoke exposure from their child. Ideally, this should be achieved by cessation of smoking. Where this is not possible, parental smoking outside the house and car, has been shown to reduce asthma severity in the child. In view of the increasing evidence that the effects of smoking on the child may start during pregnancy, mothers with a strong family history of asthma or other allergic diseases should avoid smoking during pregnancy. There are now many effective techniques for smoking cessation and parents should avail themselves of these resources. Passive exposure to cigarette smoke is clearly one of the most important and easily avoidable trigger factors for the child with asthma.

Of equal importance is the education of the child to the potential dangers of active smoking in someone with an asthmatic predisposition. Adolescent cigarette smoking rates are still unacceptably high and one of the most important determinants has been shown to be family attitudes to smoking. The ability of the child to resist peer pressure can be strengthened by understanding from early childhood that smoking should be avoided. It is hoped the increasing community awareness of smoking- related disease will make this task easier in the future.

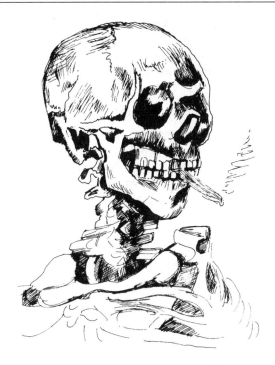

**Figure 5.2**: Vincent van Gough's 'Skull with a burning cigarette'
(The original is held in the van Gough museum, Amsterdam.)

3    Other indoor air pollutants
Emissions of nitrogen dioxide from gas stoves and unflued gas heaters, as well as wood smoke from open fires, have the potential to trigger asthma. In practice, the risks from these sources are relatively small and in most situations, the need for avoidance is unnecessary. Recent improvements to unflued gas heaters, together with the observation that minimal ventilation will significantly reduce nitrogen dioxide levels, mean that the risks are further reduced. It is important to reiterate that the most harmful and easily avoidable indoor air pollutant is *cigarette smoke*.

## DIETARY MANIPULATION

1    Food allergy
True food allergic reactions, mediated by IgE antibody, occur more frequently in children with asthma because of the association of asthma with atopy (the tendency to develop IgE antibodies). Although wheezing is a less common symptom of these reactions than hives,

colic and vomiting, children who are truly food allergic need to avoid the food concerned.

The diagnosis of food allergy can usually be strongly suspected on history, as reactions usually occur within a few minutes of eating the food. Confirmation of this suspicion can be achieved by demonstrating the presence of IgE antibodies against the food, either by skin or blood tests.

Allergy skin testing involves placing a small amount of an extract of the food on the skin (usually the forearm) and introducing a small amount into the skin by pricking it with a sharp needle. This technique causes only minor discomfort for the child, as only the surface of the skin is touched. If IgE antibodies to the particular food are present on the surface of the mast cells in the skin, release of certain chemicals such as histamine will occur, resulting in redness and swelling (hives) within 10 to15 minutes. Skin tests have the advantage that they are simple and reliable, cause little discomfort, and give an immediate result.

The presence of IgE antibodies can also be demonstrated by using blood samples, which are then incubated with the food. The presence of these antibodies can then be demonstrated by another antibody directed against the IgE antibody. This technique is called RAST (Radio Allergo Sorbent Test).

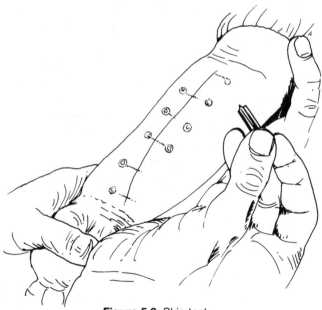

**Figure 5.3**: Skin test

It is important to realise that some atopic children may demonstrate IgE antibodies against foods but be able to tolerate eating them without problem. Thus the presence of IgE antibodies to a food should *not* be seen as necessarily indicating that the child will have an allergic reaction to that food.

Food allergic reactions occur commonly to milk, egg and peanut and less commonly to other foods such as soybean, wheat, fish and other nuts. Depending on the type of food involved, and the nature of the reaction occurring after eating the food, your doctor may either advise avoiding the food or trying to confirm the reaction with a challenge test.

A challenge test is performed by giving the food in increasing amounts over set periods of time, until a reaction occurs or the food is tolerated in large amounts. As these reactions usually occur within minutes of ingesting the food, these challenges can be done in a single day and usually supervised in a clinic or day-stay hospital setting. Challenges are not performed if reactions have been very severe and may not be needed if the food is relatively easy to avoid. They are most useful when there is some doubt about the reaction or if the food may be difficult to avoid easily.

As the natural history of food allergy in childhood is for spontaneous improvement, many children will become tolerant of a food to which they had previously been allergic. Thus re-challenge, which sometimes occurs inadvertently, may be appropriate at some time in the future.

Children who prove to be truly food allergic, should be counselled by a dietitian to ensure avoidance is complete and that their dietary intake is adequate. Children allergic to cow's milk will usually tolerate soy milk, and the majority will become tolerant to cow's milk after the first few years of life. In general, asthmatic children need not avoid cow's milk ingestion unless they are truly allergic to cow's milk. There is currently no objective evidence to support the commonly-held belief that milk produces mucus.

Other foods causing reactions can usually be avoided with relative ease, although dietary advice is essential as some foods may occur in unusual situations. For example, one potential problem for egg-sensitive children is inhalation of pavlova powder (pure egg white) resulting in wheezing.

It is a common belief that egg- sensitive children should not be given measles vaccine. Recent evidence, however, would suggest that egg-sensitive children are no more at risk from reactions to measles vaccine than those not allergic to egg, and that the risk of reaction is low. Nevertheless, it would appear prudent that *all* children be observed for a period of 30 minutes after measles vaccine.

2   Food and medication sensitivity

Reactions to foods, food additives and medications which do not involve allergic mechanisms can be described under the heading of 'food sensitivities'. Symptoms appear to be due to direct chemical effects which vary according to the substance involved. There are no simple tests available to confirm the diagnosis and therefore, a history of reaction on exposure is a very important clue to the diagnosis of food sensitivity. Confirmation may be undertaken when necessary by challenge with the substance involved. In children with severe persistent asthma, dietary avoidance and challenge may be undertaken under the supervision of a dietitian to determine whether these substances may be influencing the severity of the disease. In general, while food sensitivity has been shown to be an important trigger in children with persistent asthma, current evidence indicates dietary manipulation does not usually affect symptom severity, suggesting that it does not alter airway inflammation or airway hyper-responsiveness.

(a) *Sodium metabisulphite (223)*

Sodium metabisulphite is a preservative commonly used to prevent food from oxidising. It is thought to provoke wheezing by the release of sulphur dioxide, which is directly irritant to the airway, and in children it appears to be more troublesome when in liquid form. Other sulphite-containing additives include: sulphur dioxide (220); sodium sulphite (221); sodium bisulphite (222) and potassium metabisulphite (224).

Sodium metabisulphite most often appears in liquid form in preservative-containing fruit juices, wine, pickles (pickled onions) and in fresh salads or fruit salads offered in restaurants. Other foods containing metabisulphite include: dried fruit and vegetables; sausages or frankfurters; potato chips and other snack foods.

As reactions occur usually within minutes of ingestion (particularly with liquid forms) it is relatively easy to document asthmatic children who are sensitive to metabisulphite. In this situation, foods containing metabisulphite or other sulphite-containing additives should be avoided.

(b) *Monosodium Glutamate (MSG) (621)*

Although MSG has been documented as a cause of wheezing in adults with asthma, its role in provoking asthma in childhood is less clear. Reactions to MSG may occur several hours after ingestion, making documentation more difficult.

MSG occurs in a variety of foods such as: tomato; mushroom; certain cheeses; soy sauce; yeast extracts and meat extracts. It is also used as a flavour enhancer, particularly in Oriental cooking. Reactions have generally been described in association with Chinese restaurant meals but Italian cooking may also contain a large amount of MSG. Challenges may be performed if reactions to MSG are suspected, but this is unlikely to be necessary in childhood.

(c) *Aspirin*

Aspirin sensitivity has been well documented in children with asthma and occurs in about 20 per cent of those with persistent asthma.

It would seem prudent to avoid aspirin and aspirin-containing medications in children with asthma, particularly those with persistent symptoms. Those with known sensitivity to aspirin should ensure strict avoidance. Paracetamol is generally tolerated without problem.

There remains considerable debate about the relationship between aspirin sensitivity and sensitivity to salicylates, which occur naturally in a variety of foods such as fruit, vegetables and beverages. Current evidence would suggest that it is unusual for naturally occurring salicylates to provoke wheezing in children, even in those who are aspirin sensitive.

(d) *Other food additives*

While tartrazine (a yellow colouring,102) and sodium benzoate (a preservative, 210-213) have been implicated as triggers of wheezing, there is little evidence to suggest that they are important. In particular there has been no documented case of tartrazine or benzoate-induced asthma in childhood.

3   Prophylactic dietary manipulation

There has been considerable interest in assessing the role of dietary avoidance in preventing the development of allergic disease, particularly in those with a strong family background. Modification to the maternal diet, both during late pregnancy and lactation, restriction from the infant's diet of foods which are known to produce allergic (IgE) antibodies (such as cow's milk, egg, peanut, wheat, fish) and promotion of breast feeding, have been evaluated. There is now good evidence that manipulation of both maternal diet during lactation and infant diet, particularly in the first three to six months of life will reduce the likelihood of both food allergic reactions and eczema, particularly in the first year of life. However, there is no evidence that such dietary manipulation will prevent the development of allergic respiratory disease, namely asthma and allergic nasal problems. This evidence once again emphasises that food allergy is unlikely to be important in the development of asthma.

Some recent evidence suggests that a diet high in fish may in someway protect against the development of asthma, but such a diet does not alter the severity of established asthma.

## AIRBORNE ALLERGENS

While there is now good evidence to indicate that airborne allergens are important in the development of asthma, they are much more difficult to avoid than food allergens. Therefore, a decision regarding which children are likely to benefit from attempts at airborne-allergen avoidance needs to be made. In general, children with predominantly episodic disease have asthma which is related primarily to viral infections, and avoidance of airborne allergens is seldom, if ever necessary. Allergic factors are likely to be more important in children with persistent asthma, but in this group, the practicalities and effectiveness of airborne allergen avoidance must be weighed against the effectiveness and potential side-effects of therapy with medications. A decision regarding the applicability of allergen avoidance techniques in the treatment of your child's asthma should *always* be made in consultation with your doctor, as he or she will be able to advise you of the appropriateness, or not, of measures often advertised in the media as 'asthma cures'.

Before considering any attempt at avoidance of airborne allergens, it is important to document to which allergens your child is allergic. This can be done using the techniques described previously for documenting allergic (IgE) sensitisation to food allergens. Skin testing is probably the simplest, although RAST will also generally provide reliable results. Unfortunately, some families have embarked on costly avoidance techniques on diagnosis of their child's asthma, only to find that their child was not allergic to airborne allergens when appropriate testing was carried out. In addition, even in children who are proven to be sensitised to airborne allergens, clinical symptoms may not necessarily occur with exposure.

1    Grass and tree pollen
     Airborne pollen grains are capable of producing symptoms of sneezing and wheezing. They are likely to be most relevant in areas where pollen levels are high. Pollen grains are usually of a large size and are more likely to be trapped in the nose than to be inhaled into the lung. However, smaller components released from the pollen grains are more likely to enter the lung and it is these components that may be responsible for pollen-induced wheezing. (For example, 'thunderstorm'-induced asthma.)

     There are major difficulties avoiding pollen allergens as they are wind-borne and can travel over many kilometres. Avoidance of situations such as freshly mown grass or bush walks in the pollen season may be necessary in children who are clearly pollen sensitive. Although manoeuvres such as keeping windows and doors closed during the pollen season may help to reduce the pollen load, it is clear that it is difficult to reduce pollen exposure significantly, in any practical way.

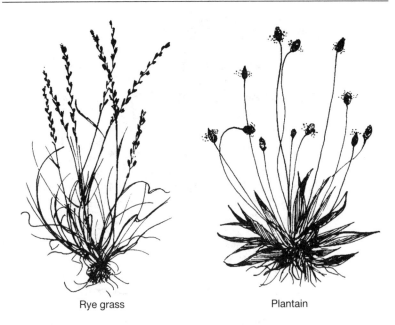

Rye grass                                    Plantain

**Figure 5.4**: Pollen allergens

2    Moulds

Moulds (fungi) are likely to be present in warm, moist environments,
similar to conditions in which house dust mite thrive. Thus sensitisation
to these two types of allergen often occur together. Airborne spores
from the moulds may enter the airway and potentially cause asthma,
although the relative importance of these allergens requires further
investigation.

Avoidance of mould is difficult, particularly in humid environments.
Reduction in mould growth can be achieved by ensuring good
ventilation and attempting to reduce accumulation of moisture. Moulds
can be treated with appropriate anti-mould preparations and use of
mould-inhibiting paint may help if recurring mould growth is a
problem.

3    Pets

Allergic sensitisation to pets such as: dogs; cats; guinea pigs; rabbits
and horses can occur due to allergens from a number of different
sources including saliva, urine, various parts of the skin and also the
hair. Sensitisation to cat allergen appears to be the most important,
possibly because indoor exposure is likely to occur to a much greater
degree.

It would seem prudent therefore, in families with a strong family
background for developing allergic disease, or in which family

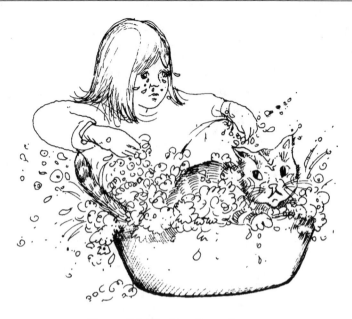

**Figure 5.5**: Washing the cat!

members have asthma, that pets be kept outside of the house. This is likely to reduce both the risk of developing (IgE) antibodies to the pet, and also the risk of exposure in children who are sensitised. Whether total removal of the pet from the home environment is essential, as a prophylactic measure, remains a matter of some dispute, but this would clearly lower the risk of sensitisation.

In children who have developed IgE antibodies to animals, a decision about removal of the pet needs to be based on the history of symptoms on exposure to the pet. If the child develops symptoms on exposure, then removal is indicated. A case could also be made for removing pets from the household of children with troublesome persistent asthma, especially if they show evidence of IgE sensitisation to the pet. However, in children with no clinical history of reaction to the pet, and whose asthma is stable, making sure that the pet is kept outside of the house may be sufficient. Recent evidence suggests that weekly washing of the cat significantly reduces the risk of exposure to cat allergen. Theoretically, this technique could be adopted as an alternative to removal.

4    House dust mite

In Australia, house dust mite allergens are probably the most important allergens associated with asthma, particularly in warm humid climates in which they flourish. House dust mites are very small insects (about one-third of a millimetre in length) which live on human skin scales. They are therefore common in bedding, carpets and soft furnishings. There are three species of house dust mite: Dermatophagoides pteronyssinus (which are most common in Australia) Dermatophagoides farinae and Euroglyphus maynei. The most important allergenic component of the mite is in the faecal balls produced by the mite and these allergens can be present long after the mite has died.

While the role of house dust mite avoidance in the child with asthma remains controversial, there are now a number of well-controlled trials suggesting that effective house dust mite control measures can reduce symptoms and airway hyper-responsiveness in the asthmatic child. Unfortunately, these trials have been done in overseas countries and their applicability to Australian conditions where house dust mite numbers are very high, have still to be proven. Many studies which have established the importance of house dust mites in asthmatic patients, have done so by challenging with aerosols of soluble extracts. This is likely to be very different from the natural exposure, as the mite faecal particles are large and most are likely to be trapped in the nasal mucosa. In addition, airborne particles are clearly likely to be more important than levels in bedding or carpet, a fact that has only recently been recognised. Thus the importance of house dust mite in childhood asthma and the role of avoidance techniques in its treatment, particularly in Australian conditions, require further clarification.

A wide range of house dust mite avoidance techniques have been suggested. The following recommendations represent a general consensus, from experts in this field of study, of the usefulness or otherwise of various house dust mite avoidance techniques.

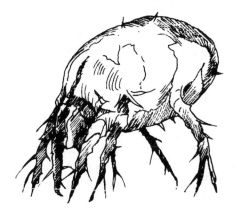

**Figure 5.6**: The house dust mite

## Table 5.1: House dust mite avoidance measures

*Probably useful*

        Moving to the Swiss Alps
        Living in an 'allergen-free' room
        Replace fitted carpets with washable flooring
        Replace soft furnishings with impermeable alternative
        Hot wash (+55°C) bedding
        Cold wash (removes allergen only)
        Encase mattress and pillow (and wash bedding regularly)
        Sun on carpets, rugs+4 hours (kills mites only)
        Anti-allergen sprays (still undergoing evaluation)

*Uncertain usefulness*

        Vacuum cleaning
        'Wet', 'dry' or steam cleaning of carpets
        Damp dusting
        Air filtration
        Air conditioning
        Acaricidal sprays

*Probably of little use*

        Dry cleaning
        Electric blankets
        Negative ion generators
        So-called 'allergen-free' products

*Source:* Adapted from E. Tovey, with kind permission.

(a) *Bedding*

Encasing both mattress and pillows will reduce mite numbers, provided that surface recolonisation can be prevented. Hot washing (> 55°C) of bedding will remove allergen and mites, while exposure to sunlight kills mites but does not remove allergen. There is no evidence to suggest that any particular type of bedding is best, provided it can be washed. Sheepskins contain large numbers of mites, and therefore are a potential source of exposure for infants, unless they can be hot washed regularly. All mattresses can develop high mite counts and therefore require encasing to reduce exposure.

(b) *Flooring*

Carpets contain large amounts of house dust mite and are therefore a major source of allergen. Ideally, hard floor coverings (wood, cork, tiles) should be used. If carpets need to be used, then rugs and mats, which can be exposed to sunlight, are ideal. Some recent evidence suggests that synthetic carpet may produce less airborne allergen than woollen carpet.

(c) *Furnishings*

Fabric covered cushions are likely to provide high house dust mite levels, although bedding control techniques are also applicable to this situation. Vinyl or leather furniture is unlikely to be colonised by mites. Damp dusting of furniture and other areas of dust collection should reduce the likelihood of mite colonisation.

(d) *Clothing and soft toys*

Both these sources are likely to contain large numbers of allergens. Soft toys should be limited and frequently hot washed. The role of clothing in terms of exposure remains to be investigated.

(e) *Control of humidity*

Humidity has been shown to be an important prerequisite for house dust mite proliferation. Simple measures such as increased ventilation and venting sources of moisture to the outside, may help in reducing humidity. Air conditioning is also effective but is expensive to install and operate.

(f) *Vacuum cleaning*

Vacuum cleaning has not been shown to be very effective in removing house dust mite and in fact, may increase levels of airborne allergen. Claims of effectiveness of expensive vacuum cleaners should be viewed with scepticism, as comparative controlled data is required before recommendations can be made.

(g) *Chemical sprays*

A variety of chemical sprays designed to kill mites (acaricides, fungicides) or denature allergen (tannic acid) are currently being trialled. Experience in Australian conditions suggest that effects are variable, generally short lived and that concentrations required cannot be achieved in some situations, for example, carpets. A decision regarding their role in reducing house dust mite allergen awaits further evaluation.

(h) *Negative-ion generators, air filters*

Negative-ion generators have no proven role in house dust mite reduction. The majority of trials with air filters have also shown no benefit.

The decision to embark on house dust mite avoidance measures will depend on a number of factors. These include:

(i)   the establishment of evidence of allergic antibody (IgE) to house dust mite;

(ii)  the severity and ease of control of your child's asthma;

(iii) the risk of exposure to house dust mite in the child's environment; and

(iv)  the likely benefit of house dust mite control measures.

It is clear that unless extensive and vigorous house dust mite control measures are undertaken, then the chances of success are small. In fact, the effectiveness of house dust mite avoidance measures has yet to be demonstrated in Australian conditions. It is therefore important that *before* deciding on a trial of house dust mite avoidance for your child's asthma, you should discuss the matter with your doctor.

5    Other insects
Sensitisation to a number of other insects such as cockroach, moth, fly and others, has also been demonstrated in asthmatic patients. Current evidence would suggest that these are a less important cause of asthmatic symptoms than house dust mite – but further studies are required. Similar problems (as were discussed for house dust mite) are likely to be involved in avoidance of these insect allergens.

6    'Allergy shots'
'Allergy shots' or desensitising injections, are designed to reduce the level of allergic (IgE) antibody and thus the risk of allergic reactions. Unfortunately, our techniques for desensitising injections remain rather crude and there is the potential for an allergic reaction to result from the injection. There also remains significant debate regarding the effectiveness of this form of therapy in childhood asthma. Our current recommendation is that desensitising injections have *no* place in the management of childhood asthma. This is also true for oral desensitising techniques (sublingual drops) which have not been shown to be of value in properly controlled studies. It is possible that with further understanding of the process of sensitisation and development of IgE antibodies, safe and effective techniques for reducing IgE levels or preventing their development will become available.

## VIRUSES

Viruses remain the most important trigger factors for episodes of wheezing in childhood, particularly in the pre-school age group. Unfortunately, with the exception of measles and influenza, effective vaccines against the common respiratory viruses are not available. Measles vaccine should be given to *all* children, including those with asthma. As stated earlier, egg allergy should not prevent measles immunisation being given. The need for influenza vaccine, which must be given on an annual basis, in the asthmatic child remains doubtful. Influenza is not a particularly asthma-causing virus, and the potential benefits are outweighed by the much better long-term immunity achieved after natural exposure to the virus. Our current recommendation would be that influenza vaccine is unnecessary in children with asthma.
    Attempts at avoiding exposure to viral infection are difficult and are likely

to delay, but not prevent exposure. Children need to be exposed to these viruses to acquire long-term immunity, and effective anti-asthma treatment can limit the symptoms which result from viral infection in a child with asthma. It is more important to allow children with asthma a normal lifestyle than to restrict them, unnecessarily, from mixing with other children in the hope that this may prevent any further episodes of wheezing.

---

### SUMMARY: TRIGGERS – AVOIDABLE OR NOT?

- Avoidance of trigger factors is theoretically the ideal way of treating asthma – but has major practical problems.
- Exercise-induced asthma can be effectively prevented by pre-treatment immediately *before* exercise or by increasing regular preventive therapy.
- Cigarette smoke is the most important indoor air pollutant and avoidance of both passive and active smoking is *essential* for the asthmatic child.
- Children with proven food allergies or food sensitivities should avoid those particular food substances, although evidence does not suggest that this will alter overall asthma severity.
- Inhaled allergens are important in the development of asthma, although effective avoidance of most inhaled allergens, apart from pets, is difficult.
- House dust mite avoidance techniques have been the most extensively studied, although evidence of efficacy has yet to be established in Australian conditions.
- Children with asthma need to be carefully evaluated *before* recommending attempts at house dust mite reduction, as only extensive and rigorous avoidance is likely to provide any benefit.
- Currently 'allergy shots' or 'sublingual drops' have no role in the treatment of childhood asthma.
- Viral infections remain the most important trigger in childhood asthma and are, effectively, *not* avoidable.

# 6

# PUFFERS, PILLS AND POTIONS

## INTRODUCTION

Ever since the ancient Greeks first recognised the symptoms of asthma, medications have been developed and continually improved, so that today we have a wide variety of preparations which can be used in both adults and children. Nearly all of these medications are modelled on substances which occur naturally, within plants or within the human body itself. In asthmatic patients, these substances are present in insufficient or excessive concentrations and some of the medications used to treat asthma are designed to re-establish the appropriate concentrations within the airways.

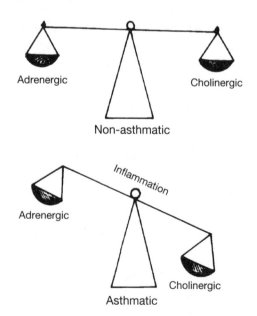

**Figure 6.1**: Balance: adrenergic versus cholinergic

In the lung there are two nervous systems controlling the size of the airway: one keeps the airways open (the adrenergic system), and the function of the other is to close the airways (the cholinergic system). When they work together, there is a balance and the bronchial tubes are opened to just the right size. In asthma, one of the problems that occurs is that the airways are more sensitive to certain triggers and the balance normally occurring between these two systems is upset. The nervous system responsible for closing the airways predominates and causes the muscle in the wall of the airway to contract, causing the effect known as bronchoconstriction (which results in wheezing or coughing). This increased sensitivity of the airways is thought to be due to the inflammation that occurs within the airways of asthmatic patients. The inflammation also results in swelling (called edema) and increased amounts of mucus inside the bronchial tubes. The inflammation is caused by the movement of a variety of inflammatory cells (some of these are called eosinophils, neutrophils and mast cells) into the airways. These cells attract additional cells and release substances which increase the inflammation within the bronchial tubes. The medications that are used in the treatment of asthma are usually divided into two groups, the first group is designed to open the airways (called bronchodilation) and therefore reverse the bronchoconstriction and relieve the symptoms of cough and wheeze. This group is often termed 'the relievers'. The other group are known as 'the preventers' as they are used to help heal and prevent inflammation and swelling in the walls of the bronchial tubes thus reducing the sensitivity of the airways and preventing episodes of cough and wheeze.

Inhaled medication has a number of advantages over oral medication in the treatment of asthma. Oral forms of medication need to be absorbed from the stomach into the bloodstream and transported to the lung before they are able to begin having an effect. They are therefore, 'slow-acting'. Oral forms of medication such as theophylline have now been developed that release small amounts of the medication over a 12-hour period. As oral medications need to be absorbed and may need to be metabolised before they can become active, they usually need to be taken in higher doses than the inhaled forms of the medication, and are usually responsible for higher levels of medication in the bloodstream and hence more side-effects than inhaled forms of the same medication.

In contrast, inhaled medications are absorbed directly into the lung, and have a rapid onset of action. Because they are only introduced into the lungs and not transported through the body to the lungs, they have fewer side-effects. Their disadvantage is that they need to be delivered to the airways by some means.

There are now many ways inhaled medication can be taken: metered dose aerosols can be used with or without a spacer device, and dry powder inhalers

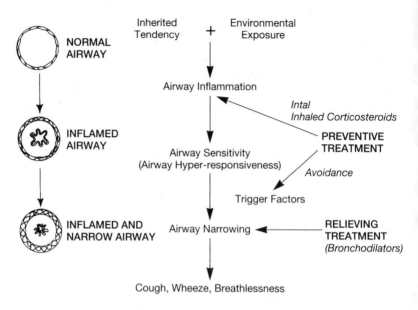

**Figure 6.2**: Relieving versus preventive medication

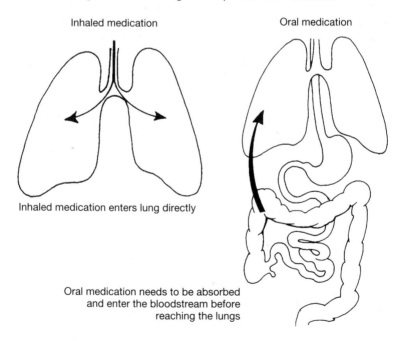

**Figure 6.3**: Oral versus inhaled medication

also provide a good alternative. Finally, in infants or in certain other circumstances (during an acute episode of asthma) both preventive and relieving asthma medications can be used via a nebuliser. These devices will be discussed in more detail in Chapter 7.

In emergency situations, some medications that are normally taken orally, such as theophylline and corticosteroids, are injected directly into the bloodstream so that they can be transported directly to the lungs without having to be absorbed from the stomach first.

In this chapter, each of the medications used for asthma treatment are discussed. In addition, newer medications which are being developed overseas (and may eventually be available in Australia) are mentioned. The final section of the chapter deals with alternative therapies and the part they play in treating childhood asthma. Although some mention will be made of the role of these medications in the treatment of children with asthma, more detailed information can be found in Chapter 8.

## THE RELIEVERS: BRONCHODILATORS

These are the medications that are used to open the airways and reverse bronchoconstriction. They should be used to help relieve symptoms such as cough and wheeze but they do *not* prevent episodes of asthma. There are three groups of medications in this category, the Beta agonists, anticholinergics and theophylline.

### The Beta agonists:
(also known as Beta-2-agonists, Beta sympathomimetics, Beta adrenergic agonists, bronchodilators)

The use of these medications to open the airways in asthma has a long history. The ancient Chinese used a very primitive form of Beta agonist made from the *ma huang* plant (which was smoked!) and in the earlier part of this century, forms of adrenaline were used to treat asthma. Since the 1940s, newer and longer lasting Beta agonists have been developed and are now available as dry powder inhalers (Rotahaler, Turbuhaler); metered dose inhalers ('puffers'); nebuliser solutions; syrups; tablets and also as injectable forms (for emergency use). When inhaled, Beta agonists usually begin working within five minutes, the peak effect occurs within 30 to 90 minutes and lasts for approximately four hours. When taken as an elixir or tablet, these medications need a much longer time before they begin to take effect. When injected in an emergency situation, they begin working very quickly. The brands that are currently prescribed in Australia include: Berotec; Bricanyl; Respolin and Ventolin.

The system responsible for relaxing the airways is called the adrenergic system. Substances such as adrenaline move out of the blood vessels (which

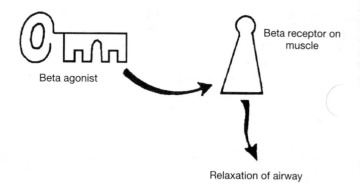

**Figure 6.4**: Beta receptor: lock and key

lie close to the airway walls) and attach to certain sites on the muscle of the bronchial tubes. These sites are then activated, causing the muscle to relax. This is termed bronchodilation. It is similar to a lock and a key, with adrenaline being a key (called an agonist) which turns in the lock (called a Beta receptor) on the muscle and allows the airways to open. Many medications have been based on adrenaline and are designed to open the airways – they are therefore called Beta agonists (the keys to the Beta receptors). Just as keys cut by different locksmiths look a bit different (but all open the same lock) Beta agonists made by different pharmaceutical companies are all keys to the Beta receptors. We now know that the Beta agonists also have some suppressor activity on the cells in the lung which cause inflammation, although this is a very minor action and they are almost always used as bronchodilators.

Beta receptors do not only occur within the lung, they are also present in the heart and on the muscles of the arms, hands and legs. The main side-effects of the Beta agonists are due to effects on the Beta receptors at these sites, in addition to the airway walls. When the Beta receptors in the heart are turned on, the heart beats faster: this is the most commonly reported side-effect of these medications, but it is a short-lived effect and has no long-term effects. This does not cause damage to the heart. Many asthmatics get tremors or shakes in their hands or arms and legs. These effects are a result of the Beta agonists working on the Beta receptors on the muscles here, although these effects are also not prolonged. If any of these side-effects begin to last for an extended time, or become more severe, this should be checked at the next visit to the doctor.

Recently, some reports have been made of a link between the continual use of Beta agonists and an increased risk of suffering a near fatal or even fatal attack of asthma. There are many theories as to why this association may exist, but for now, the precise reason for this link is unknown. It is also difficult to differentiate between an effect that is due to the severity of the asthma (thus requiring frequent use of Beta agonists) from an effect due to the medication itself. Thus, an increased need for Beta agonists or an increase in symptoms, despite using Beta agonists, should be a warning sign that an *adjustment* needs to be made to the asthma treatment plan, and a doctor should be consulted. The current recommendations are that if Beta agonist medications are needed frequently (more than two to three times per week) they should be used in conjunction with a form of preventive medication.

## Anti-cholinergics
(Atrovent, also known as Ipratropium bromide)

As mentioned above, the cholinergic system in the lung causes broncho-constriction. This system is made up of nerve fibres all distributed from one large nerve, named the vagus nerve. The most active parts of these nerve fibres are located in the muscle of the airway walls (as well as in the glands that produce mucus) and the blood vessels that lie close to the airway walls. Unfortunately, these nerves are not under voluntary control and when they become active, the muscle contracts, the glands release mucus, and the walls of the blood vessels become leaky, causing swelling in the bronchial tubes. This is what occurs during an episode of wheezing.

The use of plants containing substances that block these effects (known as anti-cholinergics) for the relief of breathing problems began in India over 300 years ago. Atrovent is the only anti-cholinergic agent currently available in Australia and it is only useful when it is inhaled. Atrovent works at the most active parts of these nerves to block the cholinergic effects, and it therefore allows the other system in the lung – the adrenergic system to open the airways. This all takes quite some time to occur and 30 to 60 minutes is usually needed before bronchodilation happens. It is for this reason that Atrovent is usually used with Beta agonists in a nebuliser or is taken with the Beta agonists from a metered dose inhaler (puffer). In some children (infants under 12 to 18 months) Atrovent, from a nebuliser or used with a spacer and mask, sometimes works better than the Beta agonists. This is thought to be due to the presence of a weaker adrenergic system (in the form of fewer Beta receptors) that is believed to exist in children of this age.

## Theophylline
(Aminophylline, Enprophylline: together they are also known as Xanthine Derivatives)

These medications have been used as treatments for lung diseases including asthma for over 50 years. It is surprising therefore, that we are still unsure of exactly how they produce bronchodilation. They do not work on Beta receptors, but it is thought they cause the muscle of the bronchial tubes to relax by some other method, probably working inside the muscle fibres. In addition to a bronchodilator action, theophylline inhibits some of the inflammatory cells within the lung; it helps move the mucus up and out of the lungs and it may increase the amount of naturally- occurring adrenaline moving from the blood vessels to the bronchial tubes. In some areas, injected theophylline (also known as aminophylline) is used intravenously as an emergency treatment for an asthma attack. In this case, theophylline decreases the amount of work that the body has to do to breathe, it helps to keep the heart pumping strongly and it also makes sure that the brain keeps sending messages to the lungs to breathe, even when it is very difficult to do so.

The most common side-effect of theophylline and the major reason that its use is discontinued, is the gastric upsets it may cause in children. The amount of acid in the stomach is increased, which may lead to nausea, vomiting, cramps and loss of appetite. Another side effect that is often reported by parents is increased activity and energy in their children. This sometimes causes a decrease in the amount of sleep the child receives and in very severe cases has been reported to lead to disruption to the child's schooling. Side-effects less frequently reported in children are headaches and an increased passing of urine. Caffeine is also a Xanthine Derivative, so the side-effects experienced by children taking theophylline are similar to the effects produced by a large intake of coffee in adults. As with any form of medication, side-effects that interfere with the normal day- to- day life of the child should be reported to the doctor so that an adjustment may be made to the treatment plan to stop these problems re-occurring.

There are two very special interactions that may occur with the use of theophylline.

The first of these occurs with the antibiotic erythromycin (EES, Eryc, Erythrocin, E-Mycin) which is often used to treat chest infections. If the child is being prescribed a medication for a chest infection, it is important to make sure that both of these medications are not taken together, without the doctor being aware of this fact. Erythromycin makes the theophylline more active, but it usually takes about six days of treatment before any effects are noticed.

Second, smoking decreases the activity of theophylline and sometimes a higher dose is needed for the control of asthma. As *no* asthmatic should smoke, this problem should not normally arise, but adolescents often try smoking and unfortunately, some continue to practise this habit and an adjustment to the dose of theophylline may be needed if symptoms increase, and the patient is unwilling to cease smoking.

Theophylline is available in many different forms, although none are inhaled. This therefore means, that as with other oral medications, theophylline does not result in immediate relief of cough and wheeze. Various strengths of tablets, capsules and syrups are manufactured and are marketed under the names Austyn, Cardophyllin, Choledyl, Elixophylline, Neulin, Slo-Bid and Theo-Dur. Some of the capsules contain granules which can be sprinkled on to soft food such as apple sauce, custard or yoghurt. These sprinkles have the advantage that children can quite often be coaxed into a mouthful of these foods, without being aware of the taste of the theophylline. Many of the currently available forms of this medication release small amounts of theophylline over a 12-hour period. They are known as slow release forms (often abbreviated as SR) and are particularly good for night-time symptoms, allowing the child a full night's sleep.

## THE PREVENTERS

Preventive medication is used as part of an asthma management plan in children who experience frequent symptoms of asthma. They are used to help heal and prevent inflammation and swelling in the walls of the bronchial tubes, thus reducing the sensitivity of the airways and preventing the occurrence of symptoms such as cough and wheeze. Preventive medication is designed to be used regularly and continuously to achieve maximal benefit. At the present time there are two forms of preventive medication in use, sodium cromoglycate (Intal) and the corticosteroids (Aldecin, Becotide and Becloforte, and Pulmicort).

### Intal
(Sodium cromoglycate)

Intal is one of the medications used in the treatment of asthma that has been developed from a plant. In the 1960s, sodium cromoglycate was derived from a substance found in the plant known as *Ammi Visnaga* which grows in Mediterranean countries. Intal is usually the first form of preventive medication prescribed by physicians for children: this is because it is very effective in many children and has few, if any, side-effects. Although the way in which Intal helps prevent asthmatic symptoms is still not fully understood, it is thought to work by inhibiting the movement of some of the inflammatory cells (especially eosinophils) into the airways. In addition, it prevents the inflammatory cells that are already present in the lung from releasing substances which increase inflammation and lead to the swelling and increased sensitivity that is characteristic of the lungs of asthmatic patients. Intal is also very effective as a preventive agent for exercise-induced asthma, cold air-induced asthma and also the development of symptoms after the ingestion of aspirin or sodium metabisulphite by patients sensitive to these substances. Intal is *not* an effective agent for relieving an acute episode of asthma: it prevents episodes from occurring.

Inhalation of a dose of Intal before playing sport or being exposed to many trigger factors often prevents symptoms from occurring, but to obtain the best effects, it needs to be taken regularly. The original form of Intal needs to be taken at least three times per day, but the recent release in Australia of a higher dose form of Intal (Intal Forte, which contains five times the dose of sodium cromoglycate in each puff) has made it possible for this medication to be taken twice daily. Intal may require a relatively long period (at least six weeks) before its effectiveness becomes obvious, and it should be commenced when the child is 'well'.

Intal is only effective when inhaled and is available in a range of devices for inhalation. Premeasured ampoules are available for use in the nebuliser, it can also be taken as a dry powder from a capsule via a Spinhaler, or in a metered dose inhaler (puffer) which can also be used with a spacer. Intal Forte is in a metered dose inhaler form. The only side effect produced by Intal is an irritation of the throat which causes coughing after administration of the medication. This usually occurs with the dry powder forms of Intal (for use in Spinhaler) and the use of a metered dose inhaler and a spacer may alleviate this problem. Children will often complain about the bitter taste of Intal: again, these complaints occur less frequently when a metered dose inhaler with or without a spacer is used.

## Corticosteroids

In 1950, it became obvious that administration of cortisone to asthmatic patients had a dramatic beneficial effect. This was of great importance, as cortisone is a derivative of cortisol, a naturally-occurring hormone within the human body. Both cortisone and cortisol have short lasting effects, so over the past 40 years, corticosteroids that last for an extended time, and with fewer side-effects, have been developed.

There are two different forms of corticosteroids used in the treatment of asthma, one form is inhaled and the other taken in an oral form. It is important to note that corticosteroids are *not* the same type of steroid used by some athletes. These steroids are anabolic steroids and have very different actions and side-effects when compared with the corticosteroids used in asthma treatment.

### Inhaled corticosteroids
(also known as Beclomethasone Dipropionate (Becotide, Aldecin), Budesonide (Pulmicort))

The inhaled corticosteroids are now available in three different forms. Dry powder in capsules (Becotide Rotacaps) or in a Turbuhaler (Pulmicort) can be used by most children over four years of age, although they are probably most effective in children over six years. There are three different companies producing corticosteroids in a metered dose aerosol form (puffer) which can be used with or without a spacer device. These medications are known as Becotide (in three strengths, the strongest one is called Becloforte), Aldecin and Pulmicort (available in three doses). The treatment of severe asthma in infants has been aided by the introduction of a nebulisable form of corticosteroid (Pulmicort Respules).

These medications decrease inflammation present within the lung and prevent further inflammation, and hence swelling and mucus forming in the airways. They do this by decreasing the number of inflammatory cells that are available to move into the airways and also prevent the release of substances from any inflammatory cells already present. Both of these actions result in decreased swelling and mucus within the airways. Corticosteroids also inhibit factors which enhance the growth and influx of the inflammatory cells: another way in which inflammation is decreased and prevented. These medications have the added advantage that they aid bronchodilation produced by the adrenergic system.

Of all the medications used for the treatment and prevention of asthma, the corticosteroids are the cause of greatest concern among parents in regard to long-term side-effects. Indeed, these are very powerful and effective forms of medication, and although they do have some adverse effects, the most serious and long term of these are usually only seen when the corticosteroids are taken in very high doses or in an oral form.

The most common side-effects are local side-effects, that is, those that occur where the medication makes contact with the body – in this case the mouth, throat and respiratory tract. The most frequently reported local side effect of these medications is the development of a fungal infection of the mouth (Candida albicans or 'thrush'). Children will often complain of a sore throat when this organism is present. Some simple measures can be taken to decrease the occurrence of this infection, and if it does occur, antifungal lozenges or solutions (Nystatin) are very effective at eradicating these infections. As an alternative, eating yoghurt with acidopholous may prevent the need for antifungal medications as acidopholous is a naturally-occurring antifungal agent. The use of a reservoir or spacer device (Volumatic; Nebuhaler; Fisonair; Aerochamber) which will allow the large particles (which would normally deposit on the throat) to deposit on the walls of the device, is one way to prevent candida from occurring. Rinsing of the mouth and spitting is another way, which should be used with the powder formulations. The other local side effect is a hoarse voice, which is usually not a major problem in children. The risk of this occurring can also be reduced with reservoir devices or Turbuhaler delivery.

Systemic side-effects, ones occurring in other areas of the body, are related to absorption of the medication into the bloodstream. These side-effects are the same as those of oral steroids but the risk of occurrence is much lower than for oral steroids as the amount of medication entering the bloodstream is very low with inhaled steroids. This amount can be further reduced by the use of spacer devices with aerosols, or by rinsing the mouth and spitting after powder inhalation. The risk of side-effects will also depend on the size of the child and the dose of inhaled corticosteroid used. Current studies suggest that the occurrence of side-effects is unusual with lower doses (400 micrograms per day and below) but that the potential for side-effects increases above this dose.

The systemic side-effects of corticosteroids include effects on growth and bone metabolism, as well as cosmetic effects, and are discussed in detail in the section on Oral corticosteroids. Your doctor will be aware of these effects and will monitor your child for these problems, particularly if he or she is on high doses of inhaled corticosteroids.

Good control of symptomatic and troublesome asthma in children has been clearly demonstrated when inhaled corticosteroids have been used as part of an overall asthma management plan. The corticosteroids are very effective preventive medications, and although they may produce some side-effects, the control of asthma when using these medications should be of prime consideration when assessing their use in individual children. The risk of side-effects from the medication need always to be weighed against the risk of side-effects of the disease-growth failure is a well-documented feature of poorly controlled asthma.

## Oral Corticosteroids
(also known as Prednisone, Prednisolone, Celestone, Betamethasone, among many others)

When asthma is very severe, either during an acute episode of wheezing or when wheezing is persistent, the local inflammation (narrowing of the airways and mucus production within the airways) is very great. In these circumstances, the dose of corticosteroids needs to be increased. The increased swelling, mucus and narrowing of the airways often prevents the inhaled medication from penetrating very far into the lungs, so in these cases, oral corticosteroids are used. Sometimes, the doses that need to be used are quite high, and as inhaled forms of corticosteroids are not as strong as oral forms, tablets – and in very severe cases – injectable forms of these medications need to be used. Infrequent, short bursts of oral corticosteroids do not seem to have prolonged side-effects in children, they do however have short-term effects: the body's function returns to normal when the oral steroids are ceased. These short-term effects are increased appetite, weight gain, puffy face, and mood alterations.

Early treatment of acute severe asthma with oral corticosteroids often prevents the progression of an exacerbation of asthma and decreases the need for hospitalisation and emergency department visits. In these situations, treatment is often begun with high doses which may be taken for a short time, or in children with very unstable asthma, may be tapered off over a more prolonged period. These medications do not begin to work until about three hours after they are taken and their peak effect occurs six to 12 hours after they are swallowed.

When asthma cannot be controlled with high doses of inhaled corticosteroids, patients may need to take long-term oral forms of medication. The use of oral corticosteroids over a prolonged period, may be associated with a slowed growth rate and delayed puberty. However, it should be remembered that children taking long-term oral steroids have very severe asthma and there is evidence to suggest that poorly controlled asthma also slows growth and delays puberty, so growth may actually improve after treatment with oral steroids in these children. Osteoporosis in adulthood has also been associated with long-term oral corticosteroid use. This problem, in children, is less likely to occur if adequate calcium is included in their diet and exercise is encouraged. Lack of exercise, due to poor asthma control, may also produce osteoporosis.

Hypertension, the development of cataracts and Cushing's Syndrome have also been reported in patients taking long term oral steroids, so close monitoring of general health by a physician throughout childhood and adulthood is needed. When possible, these side-effects can be minimised by taking single doses early in the morning (when the body releases its own cortisol), taking doses every second day, or by taking a combination of high doses of inhaled steroids in conjunction with the lowest possible dose of oral medication needed to keep the asthma well controlled. Since the introduction of inhaled corticosteroids, the need for regular oral corticosteroids in the treatment of childhood asthma is now rare.

## NEW MEDICATIONS

There are currently three new types of medications being considered for use in Australia. Many other forms are being developed but are unlikely to be released here within the next five to 10 years.

The first type of medication being developed is a long-acting Beta agonist; the second is a non-steroid anti-inflammatory similar to Intal; and the third is a new inhaled corticosteroid.

### Salmeterol and Formoterol

These are two long-acting Beta agonists currently under investigation in this country. They produce bronchodilation for up to 12 hours and have particular promise for use by patients who wake at night needing to use their bronchodilator medications. As they block exercise-induced asthma for eight to

12 hours, their use in active children with this complaint appears promising. They will be used mainly by patients who need regular doses of Beta agonists each day despite high dose inhaled corticosteroids. Patients who do use these long-acting Beta agonists should remember always, to have an inhaler of usual bronchodilator with them for emergency use. In view of the current concerns regarding the regular use of Beta agonist medication, these medications are currently undergoing rigorous testing before being released in Australia for general use. It is likely that their major role will be in patients with severe asthma, who continue to have troublesome symptoms, despite preventive therapy.

## Nedocromil
(also known as Tilade)

Nedocromil has been shown to inhibit the release of substances from inflammatory cells which contribute to inflammation and hyper-responsiveness of the airways in asthmatic patients. Like Intal, it is also good at preventing bronchoconstriction resulting from exercise and cold air: it is believed to be better than Intal in some patients. Although it has a bitter taste, like Intal, a mint variety is currently under investigation in Australia.

## Fluticasone propionate

Fluticasone is a new potent aerosol corticosteroid which appears to be more topically active. It is currently being trialled overseas and appears to be approximately twice as potent as the currently available inhaled corticosteroids. This will theoretically allow lower doses to be used to achieve control, thus reducing risks of side effects.

## ALTERNATIVE THERAPY

Chronic illnesses such as asthma are responsible for considerable disruption to normal lifestyle and in some cases, may be life threatening. It is not surprising therefore, that patients and parents of children suffering from chronic disease may seek alternative forms of therapy when faced with long-term utilisation of medications as the main form of treatment for asthma. In addition, most forms of alternative therapy adopt a holistic approach to disease, treating not only the symptoms with acupuncture, herbal preparations or chiropractic but also using hypnosis and other techniques which may explore the psychological and social responses of the patient to the illness. It is this facet of 'alternative' therapy, as well as the attraction of a 'drug-free' life, that draws many people to practitioners of unorthodox medicine. There is however, a real danger when these therapies are used *instead* of a proven asthma plan which has determined the appropriate dosage and form of medication for the individual patient to take, when both symptom free and when suffering from an exacerbation of asthma. This is of particular importance as orthodox therapy has undergone rigorous testing before being available for use in children with asthma, whereas most alternative treatments have *not* undergone the same extensive evaluation. These forms of therapy should never be used for treatment of an acute episode of asthma, and as children are often unable to detect a gradual or even sudden worsening of their condition, the use of these therapies as a treatment for children with asthma should be approached with caution.

## Homeopathy

Homeopathy operates on principles similar to those of vaccination. A very dilute solution of a substance known to cause problems to an individual, is administered as a single dose over a designated time. As a treatment for asthma, homeopathy is largely untested. It relies on the patient being affected by only one substance, and as asthma is clearly a multifactorial condition, desensitisation to one factor is unlikely to be of any significant advantage to most patients. Some adverse reactions have been reported, even with these very low doses and therefore, resuscitation equipment and an experienced physician should be present when the treatments are administered. It is also essential that this form of alternative treatment is correctly supervised, particularly when it is a child receiving the treatment, as children may not be able to recognise or communicate the onset of an adverse reaction.

## Herbalism

Many of the pharmaceutical preparations that are used for the treatment of asthma are derivatives of plants. The practice of herbalism also utilises naturally occurring substances as treatments for a wide variety of illnesses. There are some subtle differences between preparations manufactured by the pharmaceutical industry and those dispensed by herbalists. The amount of active ingredient in the herbal remedies is not necessarily known, but is usually very small; the length of time between administration of the remedy and onset of the desired effect is not consistent and there is also the danger that impurities, most often fungi, are present in the preparations. In some instances, analysis of the preparations has revealed the presence of large amounts of corticosteroids or antihistamines.

In recent years, the Therapeutic Goods Administration, under the auspices of the Federal Government, has introduced measures to protect the consumer of herbal remedies from some of these problems. All new herbal preparations must be subjected to the same rigorous studies and tests performed on medications produced by the pharmaceutical industry *before* they are allowed to be sold in health food stores and pharmacies. It is interesting to note that preparations distributed after consultation with Asian herbalists are not included in this legislation. It is extremely important to be aware of the occurrence of some interactions between herbal treatments and orthodox medications, when taken together. These interactions may lead to a worsening of asthma and it is *essential* that the patient or the parent of a child beginning a course of herbal treatments be vigilant for any deterioration in their condition.

## Chiropractic

Rebalancing of the body's function by manual manipulation of the joints and spine is carried out by chiropractors. Imbalance, according to the principles of chiropractic, occurs when nerve signals cannot be transmitted throughout the body, due to displacement of the spine or joints as a result of injury or the aging process.

Chiropractors believe the nervous system is the centre of all body control, and interruption of neural flow underlies major disease. Although most people visit chiropractors seeking relief from musculoskeletal pain, chiropractors and osteopaths also use their treatments for the management of asthma. This form of treatment presupposes that asthma is solely due to neural dysfunction, and although there is considerable evidence to suggest that blocking the effects of nerves in the airways (by using anticholinergic medications) may aid in the relief of symptoms of asthma, neural stimulation is not the only physiological cause of the disease, and relying on chiropractic for the management of asthma in children is a very dangerous practice. In spite of this warning, it is worth noting that all chiropractors in Australia must be registered and registration is subject to the attaining of certain practical and educational qualifications. In all states in Australia, chiropractors have the equivalent of a science degree with postgraduate chiropractic training.

## Osteopathy

While adhering to principles similar to chiropractic, osteopaths believe that regular adjustment and manipulation of the entire body frame is essential for health and optimal organ function.

## Acupuncture

Treatment is carried out by piercing the skin with fine needles at certain points. The needles are inserted to varying depths, and at varying angles, depending upon the points of insertion and the condition from which the patient is suffering. Occasionally, low current electrical impulses will be passed through the needles, or herbs wound around the top of the needle will be burnt to produce heat. Recently, laser acupuncture has been introduced, the traditional acupuncture needle being replaced by a fine laser beam. Acupuncture usually forms part of a more extensive form of treatment based upon Eastern medicine. This treatment includes a special diet and herbal remedies, as well as acupuncture. For safety reasons, acupuncture should be performed by a member of a recognised association such as the Acupuncture, Ethics and Standards Organisation (AESO); Acupuncturists Association of Australia (AcAA) or the Australian Natural Therapists Association (ANTA). These organisations set minimal qualifications that must be obtained before a practitioner can be fully recognised, although the requirements vary between associations. The World Health Organization lists asthma as a disease that may be helped by acupuncture. Some of the points used to treat asthma and increase ventilation of the lungs are *Tiantu* (front of the neck), *Dingehuan* (side of the neck) and *Lieque* (on the arm). In a recent study carried out in Western Australia, active and placebo laser acupuncture was performed on a group of adult asthmatics. An equal number of patients felt better with the placebo and active acupuncture and an equivalent number felt no improvement after either treatment. There were no detectable changes in peak flow meter readings; reported symptoms; pulmonary function test result or usage of bronchodilator medication.

When being treated by an acupuncturist for asthma, the patient must make sure that needles are not inserted into the chest, as there has been more than one report of an air leak from the lung, due to deep insertion of needles.

## Naturopathy

Naturopathy is based upon the premise that the body will heal itself if stimulated in an appropriate manner. Illness and disease occur when the body is in a weakened state, induced by the accumulation of toxins, exhaustion and stress or a deficient diet. The natural healing power of the body is restored by cleansing the body, relieving stress and the addition of certain vitamins and minerals to the diet.

Naturopathy quite often includes other alternative treatments including herbalism, chiropractic, homeopathy and acupuncture. As with all the other modes of treatment discussed previously, naturopathy should not be used instead of a proven asthma management plan, and should never be used to alleviate an acute episode of asthma.

Other alternative treatments:

(a) Hypnosis, breathing exercises and Yoga

These techniques may be beneficial to some patients. When suffering from an acute episode of asthma, many patients understandably become quite anxious, and this often leads to hyper-ventilation (increased rate of breathing) and a worsening of their condition. These treatments instruct patients in methods of relaxation. The ability to relax when symptoms increase, instead of becoming anxious, may prevent the worsening of an acute episode of asthma.

(b) Balanced volitional breathing

This technique involves an adjustment to breathing patterns (by decreasing deep breathing) to attain an 'optimal $CO_2$ level'. While it is known that an increase in $CO_2$ within the lung can produce a slight bronchodilation, this method of treatment is based upon the premise that asthma is solely due to bronchoconstriction. Asthma is an inflammatory disease within the airways, and the airways of asthmatic patients are more sensitive to constricting agents: it is *not* solely a condition where the airways are constricted.

In spite of a claimed success rate of 92 per cent (reduction or elimination of the intake of medication for asthma) and 100 000 Russian patients undertaking balanced volitional breathing over the last six years, there have been no publications in recognised medical journals of any improvement in asthmatic patients or any controlled trials of this technique to date.

(c) 'Salt mine' environments

This new form of asthma therapy which involves sitting in a salt-filled chamber, is now being offered in Sydney. In the late 1960s, reports were first made of a decrease in symptoms experienced by asthmatic workers in salt mines in Europe. At present, as well as at the time of publication of these reports, it was suggested that this beneficial effect may have been unrelated to the presence of salt and rather be attributable to a prolonged period in an allergen-free environment. Until careful and controlled scientific testing of these chambers have been carried out, and until a significant improvement in the condition of asthmatic patients has been demonstrated, the usefulness of this form of therapy cannot be assessed.

## SUMMARY: PUFFERS, PILLS AND POTIONS

- The use of plants and plant derivatives in the treatment of asthma has a long history. They are continually being improved and today, there is a wide variety of treatments available.
- The orthodox medications used to treat asthma can be divided into two categories:
  1 the 'relievers', designed to open the airways;
  2 the 'preventers', used to help heal and prevent inflammation and swelling in the lung.
- The 'relievers' include the Beta agonists, the theophyllines and anticholinergic medications and they all work towards opening the airways, which is known as bronchodilation. The way in which bronchodilation occurs differs for each of these medications.
- The 'preventers' include Intal and inhaled corticosteroids. These forms of treatment are used to decrease the inflammation and swelling that occurs within the airways of asthmatic children. They should never be used alone to relieve an acute attack of asthma.
- It is recommended that children requiring frequent use of bronchodilators should be using a form of preventive medication.
- Oral corticosteroids are used in the treatment of acute episodes of asthma, but are now rarely used as a regular medication. Infrequent short courses of oral corticosteroids prescribed to help children recover from an acute episode of asthma, do not have prolonged effects.
- Medications which can be inhaled produce their effects in a shorter time than those which are swallowed, and also have fewer side-effects. Sometimes, in an emergency situation, asthma medications are given directly into the veins so that they are able to begin working almost immediately.
- Although homeopathy, herbalism, chiropractic, acupuncture and naturopathy have all been used as treatments for asthma, there is no clear evidence that they result in fewer symptoms, better lung function or a decreased usage of orthodox medications in asthmatic patients. These forms of therapy should never be used as treatment for an acute attack of asthma in children, as children are generally unable to detect and communicate a sudden worsening of their symptoms.
- Similarly, while yoga and hypnosis may be useful for training asthmatic patients to relax when suffering from an episode of asthma, they should not be used in emergency situations as the only form of therapy.

# 7

# INHALATION DEVICES

## INTRODUCTION

Choosing the most appropriate method by which to deliver asthma medication is important. There are two methods by which medications are able to be delivered at home: orally or by inhalation. Inhalation of the medication is the most ideal route of delivery for several reasons:

(i) medication is delivered directly to the airways and is thus more effective;

(ii) the action of the medication is more immediate;

(iii) the inhaled route allows lower doses to be used which, in turn, reduces the potential for side-effects.

There is an enormous and ever-increasing range of inhalation devices available. Thus, choosing the most appropriate device will not only optimise the treatment prescribed, but also allow the child to take a greater part in the co-management of his or her condition. This can increase confidence and reduce the possibility of non-compliance.

There are a number of factors that need to be considered when determining the type of inhalation device which is used.

These include:

(i) the age of the child and ability to use the device;

(ii) the method by which the medication is available;

(iii) social issues such as body image and current trends.

Methods by which medications may be inhaled include:

(a) Dry powder from a breath-activated device such as the Turbuhaler, Rotahaler or Spinhaler

(b) Metered Dose Inhalers with or without spacer attachments. These are more often referred to as 'puffers'

(c) Nebulised through either a facemask or mouthpiece.

## CHOOSING A DELIVERY SYSTEM

1    The first factor to be considered when choosing the delivery device is the various methods by which a particular medication can be delivered. Table 7.1 provides a summary of the mode of delivery for each medication.

**Table 7.1:** Delivery modes available

| Medication | Nebuliser | MDI | Dry powder | Oral |
|------------|-----------|-----|------------|------|
| Ventolin | ● | ● | Rotahaler | Syrup/tablets |
| Respolin | ● | Autohaler | | |
| Bricanyl | ● | ● | Turbuhaler | Syrup |
| Berotec | ● | ● | | |
| Atrovent | ● | ● | | |
| Intal | ● | ● | Spinhaler | |
| Intal Forte | | ● | | |
| Becotide 50 | | ● | Rotahaler | |
| Becotide 100 | | ● | | |
| Becloforte | | ● | | |
| Pulmicort | ● | ● | Turbuhaler | |
| Prednisolone | | | | Syrup/tablets |

2    The age of the child and the ability to use the device are other very important factors to be considered. Table 7.2 shows the age by which most children are able to use the various devices.

**Table 7.2:** Age and ability to use devices

| | | | | | Age | | | | | |
|---|---|---|---|---|---|---|---|---|---|---|
| 0 | 1 | 2 | 3 | 4 | 5 | 6 | 7 | 8 | 9 | 10 |

|------------------------------------------------- Nebuliser ---------------------------------------------------|

| ---Small Volume Spacer -------|------------------------ Small Volume Spacer -----------------------|
          with Mask                                                 with Mouthpiece
   (AeroChamber/Breath-A-Tech)                          (AeroChamber/Breath-A-Tech)

             |-------------- Large Volume Spacer with Mouthpiece -------------|
                                    (Volumatic/Nebuhaler/Fisonair)

                      |----? effectiveness-----|----------- Dry Powder -------------|
                                              (Turbuhaler/Rotahaler/Spinhaler)

                                     |------- Metered ----|
                                           Dose Inhaler

The ability of the child to use the device correctly should be considered when choosing a delivery device. Studies indicate that many children do not use the correct technique. Often, without supervision or regular checking, the child develops a poor technique. For this reason, children's techniques should be checked, and corrected, at regular intervals when reviewed by the doctor.

3    To improve compliance and simplify the management, it is beneficial if the different medications prescribed can be delivered in the same manner. For example, use a metered dose inhaler for both the 'reliever' and the 'preventive' medication or alternatively a Turbuhaler. Again, it should be noted that not all devices are available for all medications. Each inhalation device has advantages and disadvantages. The following information describes the devices, their directions for use and the advantages and disadvantages of each.

Your doctor will advise you which delivery device he or she feels is most appropriate to treat your child's asthma, but it is important to ensure that *you* and your *child* are also happy with the delivery system being used.

## DRY POWDERS

### (a) Rotahaler

The Rotahaler is a breath-activated device into which capsules are loaded by the child or parent. The Rotahaler is designed for use with either Ventolin or Becotide rotacaps. A child can be taught to use this device at approximately four years of age but optimal delivery is probably not achieved until six years of age.

*Advantages of the Rotahaler include:*
(i)   size: able to be carried by the child in a pocket;
(ii)  ability to tell when the medication has been dispensed.

*Disadvantages of the Rotahaler include:*
(i)   capsules often melt in the heat or become moist in humid weather, providing a problem in summer;
(ii)  medication is easily tipped out of the Rotahaler if not held correctly, or the child inadvertently blows into the device;
(iii) can be difficult to use during an acute attack (unable to generate fast enough inhalation);
(iv)  can cause child to cough after inhalation, due to impact of powder in the back of the throat;
(v)   contains lactose powder and therefore, unable to be used by lactose-intolerant children.

## How to use the Rotahaler

Figure 7.1 shows how to use the Rotahaler. Common mistakes made with the use of the Rotahaler include: not holding the Rotahaler level when breaking the capsule – raising to the mouth; and during inhalation, blowing out through the Rotahaler.

1   With the light-coloured body uppermost (vertical), hold the Rotahaler by the mouthpiece. With the other hand, turn the body as far as it will go in either direction.

2   Remove a Rotacap from its foil and push it firmly, clear end first, into the raised 'square' hole so that the tip of the Rotacap's end is flush with the raised 'square' hole. This will force any previously used Rotacap shell into the Rotahaler.

3   Holding the Rotahaler level (horizontal), turn the coloured body with a firm movement, as far as it will go in the opposite direction, to open the Rotacap.

   *Note:*   It is essential that you keep the Rotahaler horizontal until you have inhaled the dose, as turning it will cause the contents of the Rotacap to fall out.

4   Breathe out until your lungs are comfortably empty. Keep the Rotahaler level, raise it to your mouth. Grip the dark mouthpiece between your

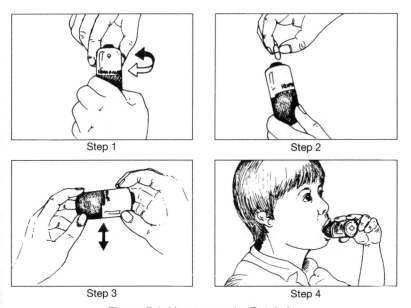

Step 1    Step 2

Step 3    Step 4

**Figure 7.1**: How to use the Rotahaler

teeth and lips and tilt your head slightly backwards. Breathe in as strongly and as deeply as you can. Hold your breath and remove the Rotahaler from your mouth before breathing out gently. You may take additional inhalations if a quantity of powder remains in the Rotahaler.

*Note:* (i) it is important to instruct the child to rinse the mouth after using Becotide to prevent the possibility of thrush. This can be attended by either brushing the teeth or rinsing and spitting;

(ii) a multi-dose (eight doses) inhaler (Diskhaler) is available overseas for Ventolin and Becotide delivery, but has not yet been released in Australia.

## (b) Spinhaler

The Spinhaler is designed for use with Intal Spincaps. Like the Rotahaler, the Spinhaler can be used by children from the age of four, but optimal delivery is probably not achieved until six years of age. Figure 7.2 shows how to use the Spinhaler.

*Advantages of the Spinhaler include:*
(i)   easy and quick to use;
(ii)  able to determine when the medication has been dispensed.

*Disadvantages of the Spinhaler include:*
(i)   bitter aftertaste – can lead to non-compliance;
(ii)  some children find difficulty depressing the outer grey ring to break the capsule;
(iii) can cause the child to cough, post inhalation, due to impact of powder in the back of the mouth.

## How to use the Spinhaler

1   Hold the Spinhaler upright, with the mouthpiece pointing downwards, then unscrew the body.

2   Check that the propeller is on its spindle, then firmly push an Intal Spincap (coloured end downwards) into the cup of the propeller. Make sure that the propeller spins easily and then screw the body tightly back on to the mouthpiece.

3   Still holding the Spinhaler upright, slide the outer sleeve down as far as it will go, and then back up again. This pierces the Spincap and makes it ready for use. This step may be repeated a second time for optimal piercing.

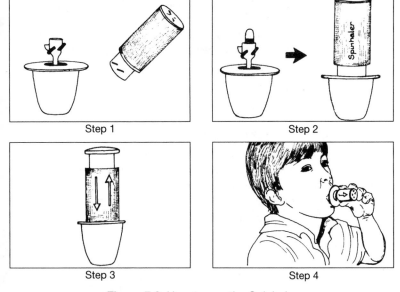

| Step 1 | Step 2 |

| Step 3 | Step 4 |

**Figure 7.2**: How to use the Spinhaler

4    Breathe out gently. Place the mouthpiece between your teeth, and tilt
     your head slightly back. Breathe in as deeply as you can. Remove the
     Spinhaler from your mouth, then breathe out gently. You may take
     additional inhalations, if required.

(c) Turbuhaler

The Turbuhaler is a breath-activated multi-dose inhaler. Children as
young as four can be taught to use this device, although recent evidence
would suggest that the Turbuhaler is most effective in children over the
age of six. Children between four and six, achieve optimal medication
delivery using a large volume spacer (Volumatic, Nebuhaler, Fisonair).
Figure 7.3 shows how to use the Turbuhaler. It is important to ensure
that the medication in the Turbuhaler is loaded with the Turbuhaler in
the upright position.

*Advantages of the Turbuhaler include:*
(i)   small – able to be carried by the child in a pocket;
(ii)  one device – no need to carry capsules;
(iii) easy to use;
(iv)  little impact and taste left in mouth;
(v)   contains only medication (no additives).

*Disadvantages of the Turbuhaler include:*
(i)   must be held upright whilst twisting the grip;
(ii)  potential for oral thrush and absorption of medications with inhaled corticosteroids. This can be reduced by rinsing and spitting after use.

How to use the Turbuhaler

**1**   **Remove the cap**. Unscrew the cap and lift it off.

**2**   **Twist the grip to the right, then the left**. Hold the Turbuhaler upright and turn the grip to the right as far as it will go. Then twist the grip back again, to the left, until it clicks.

It is important to ensure that the medication in the Turbuhaler is loaded with the Turbuhaler in the upright position.

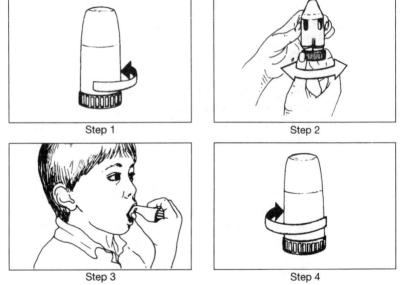

Step 1

Step 2

Step 3

Step 4

**Figure 7.3**: How to use the Turbuhaler

**3**   **Breathe in**. Breathe out gently. Put the mouthpiece of the Turbuhaler between your lips and breathe in forcefully, and deeply, through your mouth. If more than one dose is required repeat steps 2 and 3.

**4**   **Replace the cap**. Replace the cap and screw it shut.

*Note:* A handgrip is available which can be placed on the base of the Turbuhaler to allow easier rotation of the grip.

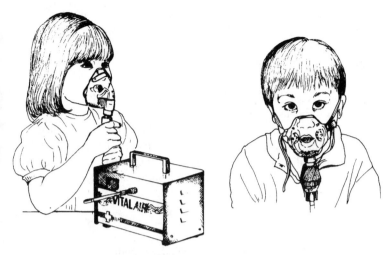

**Figure 7.4**: Using the Nebuliser

## NEBULISERS

Nebulisers are a popular method for the delivery of medication and can be used by people of all ages. A Nebuliser is a small pump that takes in air and changes the medication from a solution to a mist of fine droplets, which can be inhaled. To deliver the medication to the child, a mask or mouthpiece, nebuliser bowl and tubing are attached to the nebuliser pump (*see* Figure 7. 4). Medication is placed in the nebuliser bowl.

There are a number of nebuliser pumps available. Considerations as to the type of pump purchased should be determined by the frequency of use and the flow rate which the nebuliser delivers. To optimise nebuliser output, the air flow rate should ideally be between six to eight litres per minute. The majority of nebuliser pumps available are suitable for use for short periods (such as during an attack). However, for prolonged everyday use, it is advisable to purchase a nebuliser pump that is more durable. These include the Vitalair, CR 60 and Pulmo Aide.

The introduction of prepackaged medication vials such as Ventolin nebules, Bricanyl and Pulmicort respules, and Atrovent unit dose vials (UDVs) has been of benefit as this takes away the need to draw up the medication. This is of particular benefit to people who do not use the nebuliser regularly (child care workers and grandparents) and people with limited vision.

*Advantages of Nebuliser delivery include:*
(i) no co-ordination is required by the child during the procedure. Therefore, it is able to be used by those children unable to use other devices, for example, children with developmental disabilities;

(ii) ability to deliver a number of medications at the same time;

(iii) the use of premeasured medication vials allows ease of dispensing and use.

*Disadvantages of Nebuliser delivery include:*

(i) time consuming;

(ii) most common, affordable brands require access to power;

(iii) more expensive than other delivery devices;

(iv) optimal nebuliser delivery is dependent on mouth (rather than nose) breathing, adequate volume fill, good pump output (flow rate) and the nebuliser unit being in good working order;

(v) percentage of medication delivered is actually less than spacer or Turbuahaler delivery.

## How to use the Nebuliser

1   Gather all required equipment: nebuliser pump; tubing; nebuliser bowl; facemask or mouthpiece, and medication.

2   Ensure that the nebuliser bowl is empty.

3   If using prepackaged medication vials (Nebules, Respules or UDV) detach one of the vials. Hold the top of the vial and twist the body, to open.

4   Place the open end of the vial into the nebuliser bowl and squeeze slowly, until all of the contents are emptied into the nebuliser bowl.

5   Assemble the nebuliser bowl and attach the mouthpiece/facemask and the tubing, as directed by the manufacturers' instruction.

6   Prepare the child and start the nebuliser. The nebuliser mask should be kept in place until the misting from the nebuliser is completed.

7   Discard any remaining solution in the nebuliser bowl and clean the bowl, according to the manufacturers' recommendations.

If using Ventolin, Respolin or Bricanyl respirator solution, the following instructions should be followed:

1   Prepare all equipment.

2   Draw up the required amount of medication and place in the nebuliser bowl.

3    Draw up the required amount of normal saline and place in the nebuliser bowl. The total volume of the medication and normal saline should be at least two millilitres (mls). Some medical practitioners increase the amount of normal saline to make the total volume up to four millilitres (mls). This will take longer to nebulise, but can be helpful (especially when the child is unwell) because it delivers a greater amount of medication.

*Note:* It is important to follow the directions provided with each medication, noting the expiry date and the storage of each of the medications. Discard any remaining solution or nebules after this date.

## METERED DOSE INHALERS

### Metered dose inhaler

The metered dose inhaler (MDI) or puffer as it is more commonly known, was the first delivery device developed for inhaled medications. As shown in Table 7.1, a number of medications can be delivered by this method. As the MDI requires a degree of coordination between actuation of the aerosol and inhalation, children cannot generally be taught to use a MDI independently before the age of eight.

Some children have difficulty compressing the canister because of the distance between their fingers, and the need to press the canister at the correct time. This can be corrected with the use of a Haleraid (*see* page 99). However, the Haleraid is limited in the number of MDI's that it can be used with due to the varying shapes and sizes of the MDI's.

Children (and adults) who have trouble coordinating the actuation of the canister with their breathing, can be assisted with addition of a spacing device (Nebuhaler, Fisonair, Volumatic, AeroChamber, Breath-A-Tech).

*Advantages of the metered dose inhaler include:*
(i)   portable – no loading of medication required;
(ii)  small – able to be carried in pocket.

*Disadvantages of the metered dose inhaler include:*
(i)   requires a degree of co-ordination;
(ii)  Freon propellant from the MDI often causes children to cough/gag. When this happens, children often cease inhaling.

### How to use a metered dose inhaler

There are two different methods of using an inhaler: 'open' and 'closed' mouth techniques. Most children find the closed mouth technique the easier.

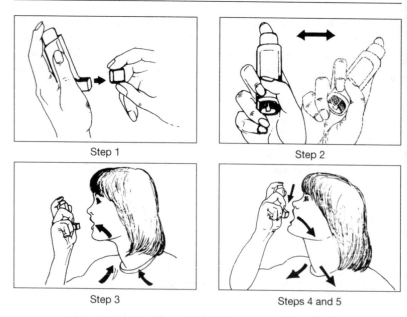

Step 1      Step 2

Step 3      Steps 4 and 5

**Figure 7.5**: How to use a MDI (open mouth technique)

*Open mouth technique* (Figure 7.5)

1    Remove the dust cap from the mouthpiece.

2    Hold the inhaler vertically and shake the inhaler vigorously.

3    Breathe out slowly and gently, until the lungs are comfortably empty.

4    Tilt the head back slightly.

5    Hold the inhaler two centimetres from the open mouth. As you slowly start to breathe in, press the metal canister down firmly. Continue to breathe in deeply. Remove the inhaler from your mouth while holding your breath, for as long as is comfortable (about 10 seconds). Breathe out gently. This allows the medication to settle into the lower airways. The breath hold is essential for optimal MDI delivery but does not appear to be necessary for optimal dry powder delivery.

If a further inhalation is required, wait at least one minute, then repeat steps 2 to 5. Replace dust cap after use.

*Closed mouth technique* (Figure 7.6)

1    Remove dust cap from the mouthpiece.

2    Hold the inhaler vertically and shake the inhaler vigorously.

3    Breathe out slowly and gently until the lungs are comfortably empty.

4    Tilt the head back slightly.

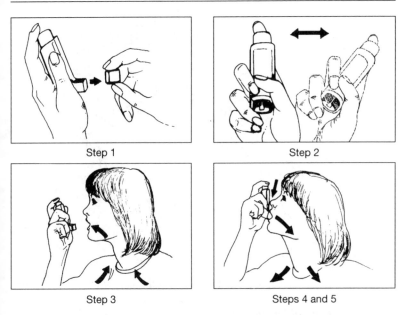

Step 1      Step 2

Step 3      Steps 4 and 5

**Figure 7.6**: How to use a MDI (closed mouth technique)

5    Close your lips around the mouthpiece. As you slowly start to breathe in, press the metal canister down firmly. Continue to breathe in deeply. Remove the inhaler from your mouth while holding your breath for as long as is comfortable (about 10 seconds). Breathe out gently. This allows the medication to settle into the lower airways.

If a further inhalation is required, wait at least one minute, then repeat steps 2 to 5. Replace dust cap after use.

*Note:* It is most important that the inhaler is triggered as you start to breathe in. If your child is not familiar with using an inhaler, he or she should first practice in front of a mirror. Escaping particles form a fine 'smoke' at the top of the inhaler which indicates incorrect usage. If more than one inhalation is prescribed, these should *always* be taken as separate inhalations, one at a time.

## Autohaler

The Autohaler (*see* Figure 7.7) is a breath-activated metered dose inhaler. Available only as Respolin, this device is different from the standard metered dose inhaler in that it takes away the need to co-ordinate activation of the inhaler with inhalation. With the Autohaler, the device 'fires' the medication when the person starts to inhale.

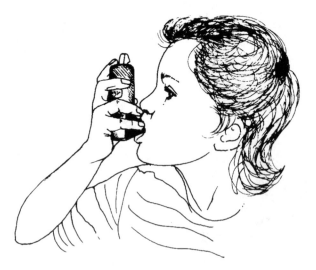

**Figure 7.7**: Using the Autohaler

*Advantages of the Autohaler include:*
(i)   requires little co-ordination.

*Disadvantages of the Autohaler include:*
(i)    lever can be difficult to push into position;
(ii)   it is important to remind the child not to stop breathing after the inhaler 'fires';
(iii)  there is still an effect from the propellant (although the amount is reduced) which causes children to stop inhaling when the medication is released. This tends to restrict its use to older children.

## How to use an Autohaler

1   Remove the dust cap.
2   Shake the inhaler vigorously.
3   Breathe out gently.
4   Tilt your head upwards slightly.
5   Place the Autohaler mouthpiece between your teeth and close lips around the mouthpiece.
6   Inhale slowly and deeply through the mouthpiece.
7   Hold breath for as long as is comfortable.
8   Breathe out gently.
9   Repeat steps 2 to 8 if more than one inhalation is required.

# SPACERS

Spacers are conical-shaped holding chambers. They allow medication to be dispensed from a metered dose inhaler into the chamber before the child is required to breathe in.

There are a variety of spacers available. Some of the spacers have small volumes (AeroChambers and Breath-A-Tech) while others are large volume (Nebuhaler, Fisonair and the Volumatic).

The Volumatic has been designed to administer Ventolin and Becotide, while the Nebuhaler has been designed to administer Bricanyl and Pulmicort, although adaptors are available to allow interchange of medication. The Fisonair, AeroChamber and Breath-A-Tech have multi-purpose ends which will adapt to accommodate a number of metered dose inhalers.

It is important to ensure that the child has a good technique using these devices and that he or she will feel comfortable with using them.

*Advantages of spacers include:*

(i)   decreases the possibility of oral thrush and absorption of medication when inhaled corticosteroids are used;

(ii)  requires little co-ordination by the child;

(iii) allows young children to deliver medication independently;

(iv)  allows inhaled medication to be delivered to very young children as an alternative to nebuliser delivery;

(v)   less expensive than a nebuliser and equally effective, provided comparable dose is used.

*Disadvantages of the spacers include:*

(i)   bulky (especially for some children and adolescents to take to school);

(ii)  the Fisonair has a soft membrane near the mouthpiece which can be displaced if the child exhales forcefully into the mouthpiece. A plastic guard has recently been designed for the mouthpiece to prevent inhalation of the membrane.

## How to use a spacer

(a)   *With facemask* (AeroChamber with mask, Breath-A-Tech with mask) (*see* Figure 7.8)

1   Assemble spacer where necessary.

2   Remove the inhaler dust cap.

3   Shake the inhaler vigorously.

4   Insert the inhaler upright into the spacer.

5   Place the mask over the child's nose and mouth.

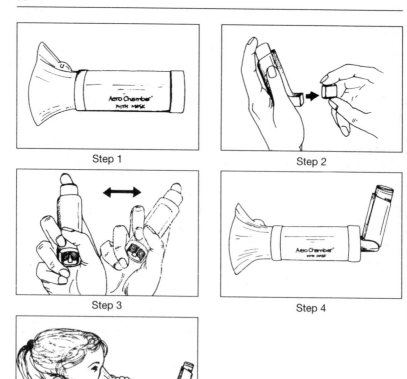

**Figure 7.8**: How to use a spacer with facemask

**6** Press the inhaler once.

**7** Keep the mask in place for six breaths.

**8** If a further dose of medication is required, then repeat steps 3 to 7.

(b)   *With mouthpiece* (AeroChamber, Breath-A-Tech, Volumatic, Fisonair and Nebuhaler) (*see* Figure 7.9)

**1** Assemble the spacer where necessary.

**2** Remove the inhaler dust cap.

**3** Shake the inhaler vigorously.

**4** Insert the inhaler upright into the spacer.

**5** Place the mouthpiece between the teeth and close lips to provide a seal.

**6** Breathe out.

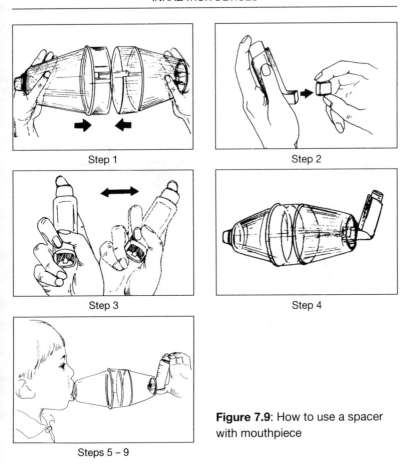

Step 1

Step 2

Step 3

Step 4

Steps 5 – 9

**Figure 7.9**: How to use a spacer with mouthpiece

7    Press the inhaler once.

8    Breathe in slowly through the mouth.

9    Hold the breath for 10 seconds or alternatively, breathe in and out gently for several breaths.

10   If a further dose of the medication is required, then repeat steps 3 to 9.

*Note:* When more than one inhalation is prescribed, these should ideally be taken as separate inhalations, one at a time. This is particularly important for preventive medication. In acute episodes of wheezing, when a large number of inhalations of bronchodilator medication is used, it may be taken two puffs at a time.

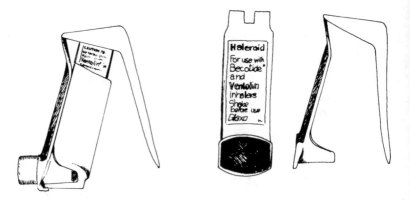

**Figure 7.10**: The Haleraid

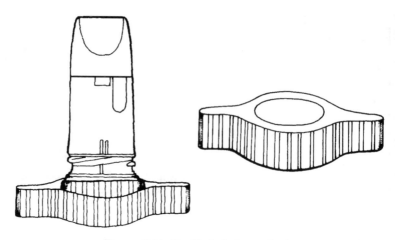

**Figure 7.11**: The Turbuhaler and grip

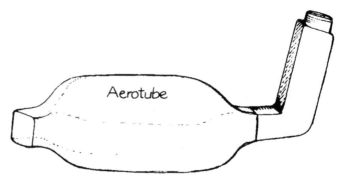

**Figure 7.12**: The Aerotube

## Inhalation device aids

### Haleraid

The Haleraid is a device which allows easier actuation of a metered dose inhaler. As shown in Figure 7.10, this device clips over the inhaler. It is able to be used with Ventolin, Becotide, Becloforte and Respolin$_{200}$ metered dose inhalers.

While the Haleraid is particularly helpful for people with arthritis, it is also useful for children who find difficulty stretching their fingers between the top and bottom of the inhaler.

### Turbuhaler grip aid

As can been seen in Figure 7.11, this device, is able to be fitted to the Turbuhaler. This allows easier twisting of the grip and is therefore helpful to people with a disability, such as arthritis.

### Aerotube

The aerotube can be placed on to the end of a metered dose inhaler (*see* Figure 7.12). This acts as a small spacing device which reduces the amount of medication from impacting on the back of the mouth. The metered dose inhaler with the aerotube is still used in the same manner as an ordinary inhaler. The aerotube is not as effective as other spacing devices.

### Cleaning

All inhalation devices should be cleaned on a *regular* basis.

The nebuliser mask; bowl and tubing; Rotahaler; Spinhaler; metered dose inhaler; Autohaler and spacing devices can be cleaned after dismantling with warm, soapy water, rinsing with water and allowing to dry. It is important to note that the device should be dry before reassembling.

## CONCLUSION

It should be noted that there are a number of factors that need to be considered before choosing the most appropriate inhalation device for a child. Careful consideration will not only improve the delivery of the medication, but also increase the child's willingness to take the medication, thereby improving compliance and self-esteem in assisting the health team in the management of his or her asthma.

With further research and development improving the devices and their mode of delivery, it is important that regular review by a health professional be conducted to ensure optimal medication delivery.

## SUMMARY: INHALATION DEVICES

- Choosing the most appropriate inhalation device is dependent on the age and ability of the child, the modes of delivery for each medication and the child's willingness to use the device.
- To simplify management and improve compliance it is preferable to use the same device for all medications where possible.
- Over the recent years, there has been a trend towards using devices other than the nebuliser to deliver medications at home. This has primarily been brought about by the development of devices which improve deposition of the medication in the airway. There are advantages and disadvantages in using each of the devices and this may influence the decision-making process.
- It is important to explain the use of the device to both parents and child, and ensure that regular checks are made to optimise the delivery technique.

# 8

# WHAT IS THE APPROPRIATE TREATMENT?

## INTRODUCTION

Before considering what is appropriate treatment, it is important first, to establish that the child's respiratory symptoms are indeed due to asthma – and not some other problem (*see* Chapter 1). Moreover, before embarking upon treatment it is essential to establish the severity of the child's asthma (*see* Chapter 4) as this will dictate the appropriate treatment. This chapter will briefly resummarise the assessment of severity, and address the standard initial approach to treatment in each grade of severity. It must be made clear that the assessment of severity is arbitrary. Thus, the initial treatment should be seen as a 'trial' of treatment, to determine the individual child's response. Adjustments will often need to be made, particularly if the initial treatment does not quickly resolve the problem. Thus, regular review of the child by the family practitioner is essential for optimum management. Any child who has asthma symptoms more than two to three times per week, which require a bronchodilator for relief of these symptoms, should be considered to have moderate-severe asthma. Such children should be assumed to have chronic airways inflammation, and therefore, must be on long-term daily preventive therapy. This can be either sodium cromoglycate (Intal), or one of the inhaled corticosteroids (Becotide or Beclomethasone dipropionate; Pulmicort or Budesonide). The use of bronchodilators (Ventolin, Bricanyl, Respolin, Berotec or Theophylline preparation) on a regular basis, without preventive therapy is not good treatment.

## DIAGNOSIS

This has been discussed in some detail in Chapter 1. It can be difficult to distinguish recurrent viral bronchitis from asthma presenting as recurrent/persistent cough, rather than as classical wheeze and shortness of breath. Under these circumstances, a provisional diagnosis of asthma may be made, and a trial of anti-asthma therapy commenced, as a diagnostic aid in the first instance. To reiterate, the symptoms which suggest asthma include: chronic night cough; waking at night with cough; wheeze or difficulty breathing; wheeze or cough with vigorous exercise (particularly running); a rapid improvement in wheeze and shortness of breath following administration of a bronchodilator aerosol; chest symptoms plus a strong family history of atopic disease; or chest symptoms plus a personal history of other atopic problems in the child in question.

## SEVERITY ASSESSMENT

The assessment of severity has been considered in detail in Chapter 4 and reproduced here for reference (Table 8.1).

To summarise, the following factors are important in establishing the severity of a child's asthma and arbitrarily dividing it into the three grades mentioned previously, namely:

1  Mild: (Infrequent episodic)
2  Moderate: (Frequent episodic)
3  Severe: (Persistent)

**Table 8.1:** Severity of asthma

|  | Mild (Infrequent episodic) | Moderate (Frequent episodic) | Severe (Persistent) |
|---|---|---|---|
| **Clinical history** | | | |
| Frequency of acute episodes (per year) | <6 | 6–12 | >12 |
| Interval symptoms | Absent | Mild | Moderate – Severe |
| Lifestyle disruption | Absent | Mild | Moderate – Severe |
| Bronchodilator usage (average per week) | <2–3 | >2–3 | Daily |
| **Physical Examination** (between episodes) | Normal | Normal | Abnormal |
| **Spirometry** (between episodes) | Normal | Normal | Abnormal |
| **PEFR Variability** | <30% | 30–50% | >50% |

1    Clinical history
     The history is perhaps the most important, and in young children, often the only means of assessing the severity of asthma. The difficulties of taking this history through a third party (the parents) has been alluded to, and the tendency of the history to underestimate the severity should also be recognised. The following historical features will help determine the severity:

(a) Frequency of attacks: in general, asthma is considered *mild* if attacks occur less than six times per year; *moderate* with attacks between six and 12 times a year; and *severe* if attacks occur more than 12 times a year.

(b) Severity of attacks: the severity of attacks, particularly those requiring hospitalisation or which are life-threatening, should immediately change the category to a more severe one, irrespective of the frequency of attacks.

(c) Interval symptoms: the presence of symptoms between acute attacks of wheezing, (such as night-time cough, early morning waking, exercise-induced wheezing) categorises children as having more than mild asthma and therefore requiring preventive treatment. In children with *severe* asthma, these interval symptoms are usually quite troublesome and often present on a daily basis.

(d) Lifestyle disruption: sleep disturbance, inability to exercise, school absence and repeated hospitalisation are features of children with *severe* asthma.

(e) Bronchodilator usage: the need to use bronchodilator on a frequent basis is an indication for preventive therapy. The requirements for bronchodilators more than two to three times a week categorises the patient as having at least *moderate* asthma, while daily usage, apart from during an attack, is an indication of *severe* asthma. The need for a new canister of bronchodilator less than every couple of months is thus an indicator of poorly-controlled asthma.

2　Physical examination

Children with *mild* or *moderate* asthma usually do not have any findings on clinical examination apart from during an acute episode. Thus the presence of wheeze when apparently 'well', deformity of the chest wall (pigeon or barrel chest), or poor growth are indicators of *severe* asthma. Children with more severe asthma may also have signs of other allergic features as mentioned in Chapter 4.

3　Other investigations

The role of lung-function testing in the assessment of severity has been discussed in detail in Chapter 4. It is of limited value in children under five years of age but should be performed in older children. Those children with *moderate-severe* asthma will benefit most from regular PEFR monitoring, but this can be also helpful to confirm the historically-defined severity when monitoring for two or three weeks may be sufficient. As shown in Table 8.1, PEFR variability above 50 per cent suggests *severe* disease, while those with mild disease have a PEFR variability of under 30 per cent. Spirometry, obtained when the child is well, should be normal in children with *mild-moderate* asthma and abnormal spirometry is again suggestive of more severe disease.

A chest X-ray is not that helpful in assessing severity but may be taken to exclude other causes of wheezing, particularly in young children. In children with more severe asthma, evidence of air-trapping or over-inflation of the lungs may be present. The establishment of the allergic (atopic) status by skin-prick tests or RAST may be helpful as a guide to outcome, as mentioned previously.

While there is some relationship between the presence and degree of atopy and the severity of asthma, this is of little practical use in terms of deciding the need for preventive treatment.

## Proportion of children in each grade of severity

Fortunately, most children with asthma have mild disease. The actual proportions are approximately 70 per cent mild; 25 per cent moderate; and five per cent severe (*see* Table 8.2). However, these percentages vary in different age groups throughout childhood. For example, severe asthma in the first year of life is very uncommon, whereas in the adolescent age group it appears more common.

**TABLE 8.2:** Asthma severity and treatment

| Grading | Treatment |
|---|---|
| 'Trivial' | |
|     Mild | Bronchodilator as required |
| 'Mild to moderate' | |
|     Moderate | Intal regularly |
| 'Moderate to severe' | |
|     Severe | Inhaled Corticosteroids regularly |
| 'Very severe' | |

## TREATMENT ACCORDING TO SEVERITY

The choice of medication is directly dependent upon assessment of severity (*see* Table 8.2). Although only three gradings of severity are discussed above, these are arbitrary and many children will fall in between. Thus, the other severity gradings are included: trivial; mild to moderate; moderate to severe; and very severe.

1    Mild (Infrequent episodic) asthma

    For those with mild disease, appropriate treatment is a bronchodilator used only as required. Namely, at the onset of an acute attack, and ceased shortly after cessation of the symptoms. The best choice is a Beta-agonist, such as Ventolin, Respolin or Bricanyl used by aerosol, up to every four hours if necessary. In children under the age of three years, this may need to be given through a metered dose inhaler (MDI), spacer and face mask (aerochamber and mask), or alternatively, an air compressor pump/nebuliser. In children from three to five, a large volume spacer (such as the volumatic, or nebuhaler, or fisonair) and metered dose inhaler is the appropriate choice. For children over the age of five years, a dry powder inhaler, such as the Ventolin rotacap or Bricanyl turbuhaler is an appropriate choice, provided the child's inhalation technique is good. For children over the age of eight years, a standard metered dose inhaler may be appropriate. However, this is the most difficult inhalation device to use. Oral medication should be avoided if possible, but if no other option is available, Ventolin or Bricanyl syrup is a reasonable choice. It should be remembered however, that the dose is considerably higher than the aerosol. Therefore, side-effects such as tremor, behavioural changes (especially hyperactivity) and mood disturbances are not uncommon. Moreover, the response to treatment is much slower than with the metered dose inhaler.

**2    Moderate (Frequent episodic) asthma**

In those classified as having moderate asthma, persistent bronchial hyper-responsiveness and chronic airways inflammation are almost certainly present. Thus, a preventive (prophylactic) treatment should be commenced, rather than using frequent bronchodilators. The best choice initially is Intal, in the high-dose form (Intal Forte 5 mg per puff). The dose is two puffs three times a day initially, and if the child is young this should be given through a spacer device. Once the child has been on Intal Forte for four to six weeks, and is well, the dose should be reduced to twice daily. In these children, occasional use of a Beta-agonist by aerosol may be necessary, should 'break-through' occur with the Intal treatment. This is particularly likely to be required either before or immediately after, prolonged vigorous exercise. However, Intal is also a very good medication to give immediately *before* exercise to prevent asthma.

The duration of Intal treatment in the moderate group should usually be for six to 12 months in the first instance. If it is clear that there has been six months of virtually no asthma, and no need for bronchodilators, then a trial off all medication may be appropriate. It is possible the child has now shifted back to a grade considered mild, where intermittent bronchodilator is considered reasonable treatment.

**3    Severe (Persistent) asthma**

Severe asthma usually fails to respond to regular Intal. Thus, inhaled corticosteroids are normally required. The initial dose is usually 400 to

800 micrograms per day, by aerosol, either as Becotide or Pulmicort. Ideally, this should be given through a metered dose inhaler and large volume spacer to reduce deposition in the mouth and throat, and therefore the total body dose of corticosteroid. Moreover, this is a far easier aerosol to administer than the standard metered dose inhaler (MDI). Children over the age of five to six years may prefer the dry powder inhaler, either as Becotide rotacaps or Pulmicort turbuhaler. With those preparations, it is important to rinse the mouth and spit immediately after the medication, to remove the unwanted mouth and throat component of the dose. After four to six weeks, the child should be reviewed to ensure that asthma control is being achieved. If not, the dose of inhaled corticosteroids should be increased. If the initial dose is proving successful in preventing asthma symptoms, (and ideally, objectively proven with peak flow monitoring showing minimal variability) then a trial on a reduced dosage may be appropriate. This should be done with continued monitoring to ensure the asthma remains under good control. Use of additional bronchodilators should be on an 'as required' basis, rather than regularly. If regular bronchodilators are still required, then the preventive dosage is inadequate and should be reviewed by the doctor. Thus the need for bronchodilators is one of the measures of asthma control.

For those with severe asthma, the inhaled corticosteroids should be continued in the first instance, for one to two years. If the dose can be reduced to very low levels (approximately 200 micrograms per day) then a trial of Intal, in place of inhaled corticosteroids, may be appropriate, provided there has been six months or more, with virtually no asthma nor need for bronchodilators. Again, the assumption is that the child has shifted back a grade of severity from severe to moderate, in which case Intal is now an appropriate choice.

## INFLUENCE OF AGE ON TREATMENT

1  The wheezy infant
   As mentioned previously, wheezing is a common symptom in the first 12 to 18 months of life, and most infants will not be distressed by their wheezing. In this situation, treatment is often unnecessary and in fact, may not make any difference to their wheezing. As these children become older, they either settle completely or develop more typical asthma symptoms which can be treated according to their severity, as outlined earlier.

   Some infants will develop more typical asthma symptoms in the first year of life and particularly, if troublesome, a trial of anti-asthma treatment can be justified. Again the choice of treatment should be based on the severity of the asthma. However, if response to treatment is poor, it may be reasonable to cease therapy, again in the knowledge that treatment may not be effective in this age group, and cessation of treatment may help in determining its effectiveness. Infants with troublesome wheezing should be referred for specialist review because of these difficulties with treatment and also for exclusion of other more unusual causes of wheezing.

**2     The pre-school child**
In this age group, assessment of severity may be difficult as the history is obtained from a third party (usually the mother) and no reliable lung-function measurements are possible. Considerable modification of the treatment plan with repeated trials on different regimes may be necessary in the very young, before good control is achieved. Clearly, patience is required by the child, parents and medical practitioner in this difficult age group.

The other difficult problem faced in this age group is the child with asthma where cough is the predominant symptom. As mentioned in Chapter 1, cough is an important reflex mechanism for removing unwanted material from the airway. It is therefore, often a very difficult symptom to treat as bronchodilator therapy may help the wheeze without necessarily abolishing the cough. Sometimes the use of regular preventive therapy, by reducing the inflammatory component of asthma, will appear to be more effective than bronchodilator alone. When this occurrence of coughing episodes is infrequent, but troublesome, a short course of oral steroids (prednisone, prednisolone) may also be helpful. There is sometimes a tendency to overtreat these children, who often do not have severe airway narrowing, but more a distressing symptom. On the other hand, they can often be dramatically improved with anti-asthma treatment, once a diagnosis of asthma is suspected. Thus, as with more typical asthmatic children in this age group, considerable 'trials' and modification of treatment may be needed before the optimum management approach for each child is found. Patience is again an essential part of the therapy.

**3     The school-age child**
While acute episodes of wheezing often become less frequent in this age group, more persistent symptoms, particularly related to exercise, may occur. Treatment aimed at preventing exercise-induced asthma as outlined in Chapter 5 should be instituted to ensure that exercise restriction does not occur.

As mentioned previously, it is important to encourage children in this age group to learn more about their asthma and to begin to take on some of the responsibility for their treatment. In those with more severe forms of disease, regular symptom and PEFR recording can be helpful in allowing them to achieve these aims.

4    The adolescent

As discussed in Chapter 4, adolescence is a difficult time where denial of symptoms, cessation of treatment and 'risk taking' behaviour are common. It is important to discuss the rationale for treatment with the young person and to provide treatment options which are feasible and acceptable. Both the aims of treatment, the methods of assessing severity and the treatment, may need to be modified to fit in with the teenager's expectations and priorities. Often the establishment of self-monitoring and management during the school age will help to overcome some of the problems with compliance. It is important for both the medical practitioner and parents to be sympathetic to the adolescent and help them achieve their independence, and at the same time, maintain good asthma control.

---

## SUMMARY: WHAT IS THE APPROPRIATE TREATMENT?

- Appropriate treatment of asthma in childhood depends on accurate diagnosis and an accurate assessment of severity. However, this can be exceedingly difficult, particularly in the very young.
- If symptoms are frequent and there is a need for bronchodilators more than two to three times per week, this indicates persistent underlying airway hyper-responsiveness and chronic airway inflammation. Thus long term anti-inflammatory or preventive treatment is essential.
- Intal is successful as an anti-inflammatory or preventive agent in most children with moderate asthma, but few with severe asthma.
- Inhaled corticosteroids in the lowest dose which will maintain good symptom relief and normal peak flow with home monitoring, is the optimal treatment of children with severe asthma.
- In children on preventive therapy, the need for bronchodilators should be minimal, and usually only in association with severe prolonged running exercises.
- If bronchodilators are required frequently, then the preventive regime is not working. This may be because:
  (a) the medication is not being taken;
  (b) the inhalation technique is unsatisfactory;
  (c) the medication is either inappropriate (it should be inhaled corticosteroids rather than Intal) or the dose of inhaled corticosteroids is too low.
- These principles of asthma treatment need to be modified according to age and individual needs.

## CASE SCENARIOS

### Case 1

Jason is now three years old. Since the age of 18 months, he has had frequent episodes of cough, wheeze and shortness of breath with intercurrent upper respiratory tract infections (colds). His cough and wheeze usually persist for three to seven days and he appears to improve following oral bricanyl or ventolin. Between his episodes of wheezing he has no symptoms of cough or wheeze, sleeps well at night and has no restriction of activity.

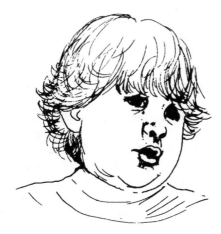

**Figure 8.1**: Jason

### What is the appropriate treatment?

Jason has episodic asthma. His episodes of wheezing should be treated with a bronchodilator medication such as Bricanyl, Respolin or Ventolin given by way of the inhaled route, using a spacer device or nebuliser.

The need for regular preventive therapy will depend on the frequency of the episodes and their severity. If episodes are occurring more than every six to eight weeks, or if less frequent but severe episodes (requiring hospitalisation) are occurring, then a trial of regular Intal therapy would be indicated using Intal Forte with spacer delivery. Provided this controlled the episodes, it should be continued till Jason has had at least six months free of cough/wheeze.

### Case 2

Sally is a seven-year-old-girl who has a history of persistent dry night-time cough, occurring around 2 a.m. and again at the time of wakening. This cough has been recurring over the last two years and has also been present after vigorous exercise. Wheeze or shortness of breath have not been evident.

There is a past history of recurring 'bronchitis' and her brother has allergic nasal symptoms and mild episodic asthma.

Physical examination reveals signs of nasal allergy and eczema but there is no wheeze on listening to her chest.

### What is the appropriate treatment?

Although Sally has never wheezed, her recurrent cough is almost certainly due to asthma. This would be supported by the signs of other allergic diseases present, on physical examination, and the history of asthma in her brother.

Although Sally no longer has discrete episodes of cough, her asthma is best described as moderate in severity because of the persistent nature of her symptoms. At her age, measurement of lung function by spirometry and peak flow monitoring may be helpful in confirming the diagnosis and severity grading.

Intal would be the appropriate treatment for Sally's asthma and should provide good control of her symptoms. If exercise-induced symptoms persisted then pretreatment with Intal or a Beta agonist bronchodilator (Ventolin, Respolin or Bricanyl) before the exercise, would be appropriate. These medications should be given by way of a large volume spacer device to ensure optimal delivery. If effective, Intal should be continued till Sally has had at least six months without symptoms – when a trial off treatment would be justified.

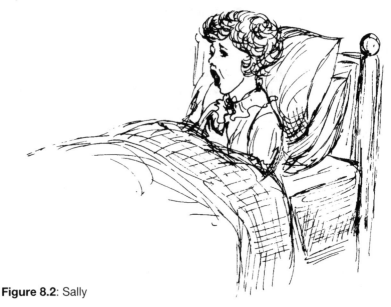

**Figure 8.2**: Sally

## Case 3

Matthew is a nine-month-old-infant who has a history of recurrent cough, particularly at night, and develops a 'rattly' chest with viral upper respiratory tract infections (colds). Although he has occasionally wheezed, he has never developed signs of difficulty with his breathing.

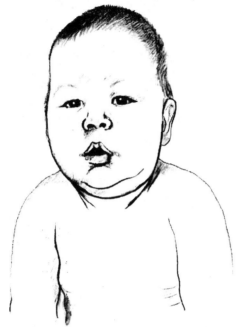

**Figure 8.3**: Matthew

There is a family history of episodic asthma in his two brothers and his father suffers from hay fever and was said to have recurrent 'bronchitis' in childhood.

On physical examination, Matthew is well nourished with his height and weight well above average. He has no evidence of wheeze on listening to his chest. Apart from some mild facial eczema, there are no abnormal findings.

### What is the appropriate treatment?

Matthew almost certainly has infantile asthma. Other causes of wheezing are unlikely based on his history and physical findings. However, a chest X-ray is probably worthwhile, to rule out other unsuspected causes of wheezing.

Provided that Matthew is not distressed by his cough and wheeze, then it may be appropriate not to use any drug therapy. If he develops occasional more distressing episodes of wheezing, a trial of both a Beta agonist bronchodilator (such as Respolin, Ventolin or Bricanyl) and an anticholinergic bronchodilator (Atrovent) would be worthwhile. These could be given by way of a small volume spacer with face mask or a nebuliser.

Matthew's symptoms may either settle down after the first 12 to 18 months of life, or he may develop more typical episodic asthma which can then be treated, according to its severity.

## Case 4

Wendy is a 14-year-old-girl with a long history of chronic night-cough and frequent wheeze, particularly when waking in the morning. On average she wakes one or two nights per week, around 2 a.m. and is usually breathless on waking every morning. She has very troublesome exercise-induced wheezing and her exercise ability has been significantly reduced because of this. She usually requires her bronchodilator puffer eight to 10 times per day and uses her nebuliser once or twice a week.

On physical examination, she is a small thin girl with evidence of a pigeon chest. There is widespread wheezing on listening to her chest. She has signs of chronic eczema and her nose is blocked because of nasal allergy.

Lung-function testing reveals evidence of moderate airflow reduction with some improvement after Ventolin. Her peak flow monitoring has shown variability greater than 50 per cent over the past two to three weeks. Allergen skin testing reveals positive reactions to house dust mite, rye grass pollen and cat fur.

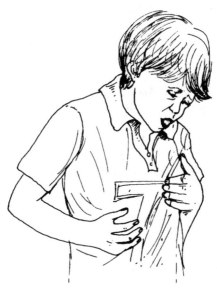

**Figure 8.4**: Wendy

## What is the appropriate treatment?

Wendy has severe asthma with persistent troublesome symptoms and evidence of persistent airways obstruction. If not already on preventive therapy, she should be commenced on a moderately high dose of inhaled corticosteroids, using a large volume spacer or Turbuhaler (depending on patient preference). The aim of the treatment would be to reduce her symptoms and need for bronchodilator puffer, improve her lung function and peak flow variability and normalise her lifestyle. Treatment will need to be adjusted according to her response and she should be encouraged to monitor her symptoms, bronchodilator usage and peak flow regularly.

In view of the severity of her asthma and her allergic background, attempts at allergen avoidance should be considered, particularly if her response to conventional treatment is sub-optimal.

# 9

# THE ASTHMA MANAGEMENT PLAN

## INTRODUCTION

Asthma is now one of the major public health problems in Australia and New Zealand. Despite our improved knowledge and understanding of this condition, and advances in the management, all available statistics indicate worsening of the problem. In particular, there appears to be an increasing need for hospitalisation (particularly in children) and a persistently high mortality rate – although most of the increase is in the elderly. It is now evident that over one million Australians have asthma and that it is one of the leading illnesses, as reported in the most recent *Australian Health Survey,* published by the Bureau of Statistics. Unfortunately, what is also clear from studies in many countries of the world, is that asthma is still generally under-diagnosed, and more particularly, under-treated. Thus, although effective treatments are available, they are not fully utilised.

## NATIONAL CONSENSUS TREATMENT PLANS

With the recognition that asthma is a major health burden, consuming large amounts of health resources, and that it is generally under-treated, various national consensus treatment plans have been devised. These are now available for Australia (both adult and paediatric), the United Kingdom, Canada and the USA. There is even an international consensus management plan which has been published for both children and adults. There is a surprisingly high level of agreement on the optimal appropriate management of childhood asthma throughout the world. Thus, it is extremely disheartening to find that these plans are not fully implemented.

The management plans are relatively simple and based on standard principles of good medical practice for any recurring or chronic medical condition.

## GOALS OF TREATMENT

The goals of treatment are simple:
  (i)   the appropriate recognition of asthma;
  (ii)  complete abolition of symptoms;
  (iii) normalisation of lung function; and
  (iv)  prevention of acute attacks.

With respect to symptoms, there should be no restriction on normal physical activity. This includes full participation in all forms of exercise and competitive sports. The only exception to this is that asthmatic children should not undertake scuba-diving, because of the inherent risks involved for those with definite asthma. There should not be excessive school absences due to asthma, nor interference with good quality sleep. Further, there should be infrequent need to use relieving doses of bronchodilators, and ideally, these should only be used on several occasions per week, particularly before or after vigorous physical activity. There should be no adverse side-effects from any treatment. Lung function (if this can be measured) should be normal, and there should be no major fluctuations of lung function on a day-to-day basis (as measured by peak expiratory flow rate meters twice daily at home). Failure to achieve these goals satisfactorily, indicates the need for revision of that individual child's treatment.

In short, the aim of optimum asthma management is for the child to lead a normal life, both in terms of quality and duration.

## The principle of co-management of asthma

Optimum management should be seen as a co-operative agreement between the patient, his or her family, the child's school/school teachers and the doctor. Although self-management is often mentioned, this is also inappropriate – as is 'doctor-dominated' management. Doctors should not be asking patients (or parents of patients) to look after this complex disease on their own, but rather in partnership with their medical practitioners.

The involvement of asthma education nurses, physiotherapists and organisations such as Asthma Foundations, is strongly encouraged.

The objective of co-management is to ensure there is complete agreement and good understanding of the asthma condition itself: the goals of treatment; the appropriate medications; their correct administration and frequency of usage; and the appropriate sequence of steps to take, should there be an acute flare-up of the child's asthma. The international consensus plan for children has identified key elements of co-management: complete understanding of asthma; monitoring of symptoms; peak flow and drug usage; and a pre-arranged and agreed Home Management Plan (*see* Figures 9.1a and 9.1b). In addition to educational material, effective co-management may entail

# Instructions for Home Management of Asthma

## (A) WHEN WELL:

**Daily medications**

### INTAL FORTE
2 puffs via Fisonair
twice a day

## (B) WHEN NOT WELL: CONTINUE INTAL

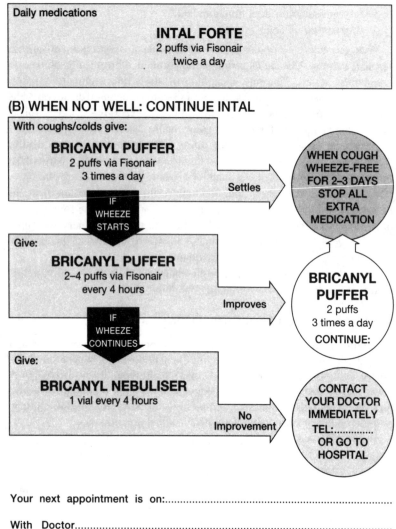

With coughs/colds give:

**BRICANYL PUFFER**
2 puffs via Fisonair
3 times a day

Settles

IF WHEEZE STARTS

Give:

**BRICANYL PUFFER**
2–4 puffs via Fisonair
every 4 hours

Improves

IF WHEEZE CONTINUES

Give:

**BRICANYL NEBULISER**
1 vial every 4 hours

No Improvement

WHEN COUGH WHEEZE-FREE FOR 2–3 DAYS STOP ALL EXTRA MEDICATION

**BRICANYL PUFFER**
2 puffs
3 times a day
CONTINUE:

CONTACT YOUR DOCTOR IMMEDIATELY TEL:............. OR GO TO HOSPITAL

Your next appointment is on:............................................................................

With Doctor................................................................................................

**Figure 9.1a**: Home Management Plan – Example 1

# Instructions for Home Management of Asthma

## (A) WHEN WELL:

Daily medications

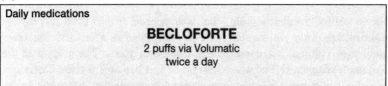

**BECLOFORTE**
2 puffs via Volumatic
twice a day

## (B) WHEN NOT WELL: CONTINUE BECLOFORTE

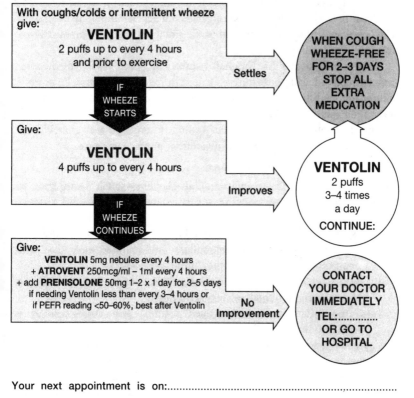

Your next appointment is on:.................................................................................

With Doctor.................................................................................................

**Figure 9.1b**: Home Management Plan – Example 2

behavioural changes on the part of both the child and the family, in terms of complying with the agreed goals previously mentioned, particularly compliance with medication regimens.

## THE PAEDIATRIC ASTHMA MANAGEMENT PLAN

The so-called 'paediatric point plan' was devised in mid-1990 and closely follows the *Adult Australian Asthma Management Plan* and the other published national and international consensus plans. The release of the Asthma Management Plan was a key part of The National Asthma Campaign, a public health exercise which was devised to ensure that this public health problem was appropriately managed.

The initial goal was improvement in the understanding of the disease by health professionals (doctors, pharmacists, nurses and ambulance officers). Thus, copies of this plan were sent to all practising doctors in Australia to ensure widespread dissemination.

The second phase of the National Asthma Campaign involved education, aimed directly at asthma sufferers, in an effort to increase knowledge about asthma and healthy life-styles, which included asthma education programs throughout schools in Australia.

The third phase of the National Asthma Campaign was aimed at the general public as a major 'asthma awareness' media campaign.

**Step1:** Assess severity of the asthma

This has already been discussed in detail in Chapters 4 and 8. To reiterate, the key questions for quickly assessing severity of an individual child's asthma are:

  (i)   is a bronchodilator needed immediately on waking, or can it wait?
  (ii)  how many doses of bronchodilator are required each day? This should be less than two to three times per week;
  (iii) does exercise cause cough or wheeze? And does it limit the ability of the child to participate in such activities?
  (iv)  is the child's sleep disturbed due to asthma – from cough, wheeze, or difficulty breathing?

A positive response to these questions will rapidly establish the presence of moderate or severe asthma as discussed in Chapters 4 and 8.

This historical information should be supported by objective measures of lung function (if possible) and the best available method is home peak flow monitoring. While this is appropriate for school age children, it is usually impossible in the very young child. It is not usually necessary to monitor peak flow for prolonged periods. However, at the initial assessment, a two week period of peak flow readings, twice daily before and after bronchodilator (if being used) is an extremely helpful way of accurately assessing the severity of an individual child's disease.

**Step 2:** Achieve the 'best' lung function

Unfortunately, most children under the age of four or five years find it impossible to use a peak flow meter reliably. For this group, 'best' lung function can only be judged by clinical symptoms and physical examination. 'Best' lung function is achieved by prescribing the appropriate medication for that severity of disease. For those with mild/infrequent episodes of asthma, the intermittent use of an inhaled bronchodilator is appropriate. For those too young to use a standard hand-held device, a small Aerochamber with mask or similar product is extremely useful. For the older child, three to five years, a large volume spacer, and for those over the age of five or six years, a dry powder inhaler, such as the Turbuhaler or Rotahaler is appropriate. If all of these are impossible, the air compressor pump/nebuliser may be required. However, this is expensive, cumbersome, and takes at least 10 minutes to deliver the dose of bronchodilator effectively. Oral bronchodilators are rarely indicated and the aerosol route is always preferred. Aerosols minimise the dose, and any potential side-effects, and gives very rapid relief of symptoms.

Children with moderate asthma (as defined in Chapters 4 and 8) should be commenced on inhaled Intal (sodium cromoglycate) on a regular basis and may occasionally need a bronchodilator.

For children with severe disease (as defined in Chapters 4 and 8), inhaled corticosteroids will be necessary and the dose will vary considerably from child to child. Again, if the inhaled corticosteroid is effectively controlling the asthma, the need for additional bronchodilators will be infrequent.

Once the child is given a trial of treatment as described, re-assessment is essential and if possible this should include measurement of lung function with home peak flow monitoring, to obtain objective evidence that the 'best' lung function is being achieved.

**Step 3**: Maintain 'best' lung function by minimising avoidable triggers and aggravating factors

In young children, the most important triggers of asthma attacks are viral respiratory tract infections, which are difficult, if not impossible to avoid effectively. These are particularly likely to occur in the winter months, especially when children commence pre-school, kindergarten or school, because of the heavy exposure they will receive from their peers. A trigger which may be important, and which is theoretically avoidable, is passive cigarette smoking. It is important that the parents of asthmatic children do *not* allow any adults to smoke in the same house as the asthmatic child.

For children who wheeze (or sneeze) on exposure to cats, this is also a potentially avoidable trigger. Cats should be confined to non-living room areas and must stay out of the asthmatic child's bedroom. Ideally, if there is a definite history of symptoms after exposure to cats, then cats should not be kept in that household. The child who is allergic to cats is actually allergic to the cat's saliva. The saliva is on the fur because cats are constantly licking and cleaning their coats.

Dogs are not in the habit of doing this, and for a number of genuine reasons, allergy to dogs is far less common.

Other avoidable trigger factors include foods and medicines. While legend has it that 'milk produces mucus' and is therefore, bad for children with allergies/asthma – the evidence for this is non-existent. Indeed, milk is a very important source of calories, protein and calcium for children. Thus, very good evidence of problems from milk must be available before this is eliminated from a child's diet.

Certain food additives are able to trigger asthma attacks, particularly metabisulphite, which is present in high concentrations in some dried fruits, pickled onions, and beverages. However, colouring agents and flavouring agents (tartrazine and MSG) appear to be uncommon triggers for asthma, particularly in children. Thus, unless there is a good history of asthma symptoms following ingestion of these products, they should not be removed from the child's diet.

Medicines such as aspirin can trigger acute attacks, particularly in those with more severe forms of asthma. For this reason, it is best to use paracetamol rather than aspirin in children with asthma.

The most important allergen in childhood asthma, particularly on the coastal parts of Australia, is house dust mite. The difficulty however, is to remove house dust mite from houses effectively, because they are generally carpeted, poorly ventilated and thus 'house dust mite friendly'. Considerable research is in progress to find effective means of reducing house dust mite exposure in homes. Outdoor allergens, such as grass pollens, can be important, particularly in rural areas and southern parts of Australia (such as Melbourne and Adelaide). However, it is again difficult to avoid these allergens. Thus, the current emphasis is on medical treatment to reverse the underlying abnormality in the airways (hyper-responsiveness or 'twitchiness') rather than avoiding the triggers which aggravate the asthma.

Although exercise is a well known trigger of asthma attacks, all children should take part in physical activity, including competitive sport. Adequate preventive treatment should allow this to be possible in all cases. For very hard or prolonged physical activity, additional doses of either Intal or a bronchodilator may be necessary immediately *prior* to the activity.

Alternative methods for overcoming exercise-induced asthma include a good 'warm-up' period and switching to sports which are more intermittent, rather than prolonged, endurance-type activities. Swimming is the least likely exercise to trigger an asthma attack.

A more detailed discussion of avoidance of trigger factors can be found in Chapter 5.

**Step 4:** Prescribe optimal medication to maintain the best lung function

The appropriate medication is based upon the assessment of severity (*see* Chapters 4 and 8). Following review, after four to six weeks, an assessment can then be made as to the adequacy of this initial treatment. Once the asthma is under good control, and the 'best' lung function is being maintained, it is usually possible to reduce the frequency of medications to twice daily (Intal or inhaled corticosteroids). Bronchodilator treatment should be rarely required as very few symptoms should be appearing. Increasing requirements for additional bronchodilator use indicates loss of asthma control and the need to switch from Intal to inhaled corticosteroids; to increase the dose of inhaled corticosteroids; or to change from inhaled to oral corticosteroids.

All medications should be given as aerosol, and the use of large volume aerosol spacers is recommended, particularly in younger age groups (less than six years) and those receiving doses of inhaled corticosteroids in excess of 400 micrograms per day. Although the concern of side-effects from inhaled corticosteroids is ever present in both parents and doctor, the risk of adverse effects is extremely low, provided the dose is less than 400 micrograms per day. Side-effects are unusual even at doses of 800 micrograms per day. It is important to remember that the use of even higher dose-inhaled corticos-teroids *is* warranted, as the benefit of inhaled corticosteroids far outweigh the consequences of uncontrolled asthma.

Other asthma medications, such as Theophylline (Neulin Sprinkles, Theodur) and/or Ipratropium bromide (Atrovent), are rarely used on any regular basis. However, these medications may be useful for acute flare-ups of asthma not responding promptly to inhaled Beta agonists (such as Ventolin/Bricanyl).

**Step 5:** Develop and write an action or crisis plan (*see* Figure 9.2)

This written plan should contain information relating to both regular preventive treatment and specific instructions on what to do – should there be any worsening of the asthma. The management of acute asthma must be judged on an individual basis, and the written action plan may be either 'symptom-based' or 'peak flow-'based, depending upon the child's age and ability to perform reliable peak flow-readings.

Included in this plan should be specific instructions on the frequency of use of bronchodilators (such as Ventolin), the dosage to be used, the device, plus when to start oral corticosteroids (Prednisone/Prednisolone), and in what dosage. Also, at what stage of the attack to call for help, either by bringing the child to hospital, to a medical practitioner, or calling for an ambulance.

No two family situations will be identical. Therefore, the medical

## Crisis Plan for an Asthma Attack

It is important to have a plan worked out ahead in case you have a severe asthma attack.

Important Peak Flow Readings:

| | |
|---|---|
| Best peak flow | 420 |
| Peak flow requiring additional medication | 300 |
| Peak flow requiring urgent medical attention | 210 |

### INDICATIONS OF WORSENING ASTHMA IF:

1. You are waking through the night with cough, wheeze or shortness of breath.
2. You have morning wheeze that persists despite usual treatment.
3. Your response to usual medication is not as good OR effect not lasting very long (i.e. you may require your metered aerosol more frequently than normal).
4. You become short of breath during the day and find it difficult to do your usual activities.
5. Your peak flow meter shows:
   – more morning dip than usual
   – lower pre-bronchodilator readings
   – less response to bronchodilator
   – a trend or pattern that is more unstable or downward.
6. Your peak flow is below 250 after bronchodilator.

If you have any of the above symptoms, CONTACT your doctor. If he is unavailable, or you experience SUDDEN, SEVERE ASTHMA DO NOT DELAY, go to the nearest hospital, preferably by ambulance.

The sooner EXTRA TREATMENT for asthma is commenced, the sooner you will feel better.

MONITOR your asthma carefully after a severe episode and always check back to your doctor.

**R.N.S Asthma Education Programme**
**Departments of Patient Education and Thoracic Medicine.**

**ASTRA**

### Respiratory Treatment Card

Name: _____

Address: _____

Telephone No:  H. _____
W. _____

Family doctor: _____

Telephone No:  W. _____
A.H. _____

Specialist: _____

Ambulance: 000

**Medication Chart** — supplied with compliments of Astra, makers of Bricanyl™ Aerosol, Bricanyl™ Misthaler™ and Theo-Dur™

| | | TIMES | | | | | INSTRUCTIONS* |
|---|---|---|---|---|---|---|---|
| MEDICATION | DOSE | | | | | | |

Regular Therapy

Additional Therapy

*Instructions for regular therapy and additional medication needed when asthma gets worse.

### WHAT YOU CAN DO TO HELP YOURSELF

1. Remember to take your medications
2. Carry this card at all times
3. Always carry your bronchodilator aerosol
4. Check your aerosol is not empty
5. Have spare medication available
6. Consider your asthma when making plans to travel

**Figure 9.2**: Asthma Management Crisis Plan

practitioner, the child, and parents, must decide exactly how far they will go in terms of managing an acute attack at home. This will largely depend upon the individual's experience with managing acute attacks in the home environment; the severity of the child's asthma; its usual response to treatment; and any past history of severe life-threatening episodes.

Fortunately, an action plan based on symptoms appears to be just as useful as that based on peak flow, and this has now been tested in a large general practitioner-based research trial in the United Kingdom. In that study, both children and adults were issued with either a peak flow-based written action plan or a symptom-based written action plan (*see* Table 9.1). The use of these home management plans reduced the need for urgent medical consultations and the frequency of severe flare-ups of asthma. The reductions were the same, irrespective of whether peak flow or symptoms were used, and irrespective of the subjects being children or adults.

**TABLE 9.1:** Action plan based on either symptoms or peak flow

| Symptoms | Action | Peak Flow Status |
|---|---|---|
| 1 None | Continue **normal** maintenance treatment | >70% of best |
| 1a Cold (flu or coryza) or feeling of tightness | Bronchodilator two puffs up to every 4 hours | |
| 2 Wheezing at night or persistent cough | **Double dose of inhaled steroids** until achieve previous baseline or return to normal; continue on this increased dose for same number of days bronchodilator two puffs up to every 4 hours. If on INTAL, switch to inhaled steroids until return to normal (as above) | <70% of best |
| 3 Bronchodilator only lasts two hours and normal activities cause shortness of breath | **Start oral prednisolone** at 20 to 40 milligrams per day and contact general practitioner. Continue to use this dose for the number of days required to return to normal; reduce oral prednisolone to 10 to 20 milligrams per day for same number of days, then stop prednisolone | <50% of best |
| 4 Bronchodilator lasts only 30 minutes or talking is difficult | Contact general practitioner **urgently** or contact **ambulance** or go directly to **hospital** | <30% of best |

Source: Adapted from I Charlton et al., with kind permission.

**Step 6:** Educate the child, family and school, and review the child and family regularly

As has already been pointed out, the overall aim of asthma treatment is to allow the child to live a normal life, by using medications optimally. This includes factual information regarding the cause of asthma; the triggers; and the mode of action of the various medications, particularly the clear distinction between bronchodilators and preventive agents. Careful instructions and the repeated checking on technique of inhalation and the appropriate device for the child's age and competence with the aerosols should be reviewed regularly. The intention of these regular reviews of the child is to ensure that he or she is achieving the goals of management, and that good control of the asthma is being maintained.

The commonest causes of failure to respond or to maintain the response to adequate therapy is non-compliance (missing doses of preventive treatment), poor inhalation technique, or a combination of both. However, if symptoms are proving refractory to treatment – and treatment is being taken as prescribed – referral to a specialist paediatrician is appropriate.

Although all parents would like their children to be taken off preventive treatment as soon as possible, there is no uniformity of opinion as to the minimum time required before cessation of long-term preventive therapy. As a general rule, if the child has been totally free from symptoms and has normal lung function for three to six months, then a trial of either a lower dose of preventive treatment or cessation of preventive treatment (particularly if this is with Intal), together with careful monitoring of the response, is a reasonable approach.

## RECOGNITION AND MANAGEMENT OF THE ACUTE-SEVERE ATTACK OF ASTHMA

This has already been outlined in Step 5. Should the child have to go to hospital by ambulance, the treatment is likely to include very frequent or even continuous nebulised bronchodilators (usually Ventolin). This is normally delivered by using oxygen from a wall oxygen supply rather than a compressor pump. Because systemic corticosteroids (oral Prednisolone) is

**Table 9.2:** Assessing the severity of attack

(i)  Mild attack
cough
soft wheeze
minor difficulty breathing
no difficulty speaking in sentences

(ii) Moderate attack
persistent cough
loud wheeze
obvious difficulty breathing
able to speak in short sentences only

(iii) Severe attack[1]
very distressed and anxious
gasping for breath
unable to speak more than a few words in one breath
pale and sweaty
may be blue around lips (cyanosis)

1 Features that demand immediate action ( ambulance), are failure to achieve more than 30 minutes relief with bronchodilators; difficulty in speaking in sentences; blue discolouration of the lips (cyanosis); or any alteration in the level of the child's consciousness (disorientation, 'passing out', marked agitation).

one of the most effective means of aborting a severe attack of asthma, this will usually be given quite early in the course of the hospital care, usually in the Accident and Emergency Department. If the child is extremely ill, the corticosteroids may be given intravenously. In some hospitals, intravenous aminophylline (theophylline) may be added if there is not a good response to the combination of frequent Ventolin, continuous oxygen and high-dose systemic corticosteroids. In some hospitals, nebulised Ipratropium bromide (Atrovent) may also be added to the nebulised Ventolin. This is in the expectation that this combination will give a better response than Ventolin alone, and obviate the need for intravenous aminophylline.

Parents should have no fear of their child taking Prednisolone in short courses for acute flare-ups of asthma. This is not associated with long-term consequences and is one of the most effective agents for rapidly halting the progression of a severe attack of asthma.

Should a child have a severe attack of asthma needing either hospitalisation, attendance in an Accident and Emergency Department, or a trip to hospital by ambulance, then a total revision of his or her usual treatment is essential to prevent a repetition of this complication of asthma.

---

### SUMMARY: THE ASTHMA MANAGEMENT PLAN

- Asthma is a major public health problem in our community. While safe and effective treatment is available, it does require a commitment from the child, the family, and the medical practitioner. For the doctor, this means prescribing the appropriate management regimen. For the child and family it means complying with the prescribed program.
- Unfortunately, under-treatment of asthma is common. This may be due to failure to recognise the severity of the disease at a medical level, and/or a tendency to cease regular preventive treatment by parents and/or the child.
- With appropriate education in regard to all aspects of asthma and asthma care, compliance with treatment *will* improve. Thus the suffering of the child will diminish to a level where his or her quality of life is normal.

# 10

# WILL MY CHILD GROW OUT OF ASTHMA?

## INTRODUCTION

This crucial question is asked by virtually all parents of asthmatic children. Unfortunately, however, it is difficult to give a definite reply. A number of factors have now been identified which allow us to give at least a statistical probability of either persistence or disappearance of asthma over time.

Excellent long-term studies have been performed in children with asthma, both in Australia and overseas, which have enabled us to make predictions about the child's future asthma. It is important to realise, however, that children who have had asthma, even though they appear to have outgrown the symptoms, are at increased risk of their asthma relapsing in the future. Thus, asthma is best seen as a condition that can go into very long remissions, rather than totally disappearing. In other words, there is a sizeable proportion of adults who remain 'latent' asthmatics. They are at risk of recurrence of their childhood asthma, should they encounter environmental circumstances which are able to trigger the redevelopment of asthma in later life.

## DEFINITIONS / TERMINOLOGY

When dealing with the natural history of childhood asthma, it is important to be clear on the terminology. The current accepted clinical definition for asthma is as follows:

In *young children,* asthma is a condition in which episodic wheeze and/or cough occur in a clinical setting where asthma is likely, and where other, rarer conditions have been excluded.

In adults, this definition is extended to include evidence of reversible air-flow obstruction (as measured with lung function). Many would add evidence of abnormal airway responsiveness (as measured by provocation testing, such as histamine, methacholine or exercise). Some would also suggest including the presence of chronic eosinophilic inflammation in the airways (as determined by biopsy of the airways).

Because children of pre-school age are unable to do reliable lung-function testing, the definition is simply based on history and physical findings. Although airway responsiveness can be measured in children over the age of five years, at present, it is very unusual to biopsy the airways of children with asthma. Therefore, we are still uncertain as to whether this pathology does exist in childhood asthma, or how this correlates with grades of severity. Until these questions are answered, we assume that any child needing *bronchodilators* more than *two or three times per week* for asthma symptoms, has both chronic inflammation in the airways and persistently abnormal bronchial responsiveness.

## FACTORS WHICH PREDICT THE NATURAL HISTORY OF ASTHMA

1    The severity of asthma
     Those with the mildest forms of asthma have the greatest likelihood of outgrowing the symptoms of asthma in early, or mid -childhood. Conversely, those with severe persistent or chronic asthma have far less chance of outgrowing their disease. Nevertheless, even this group frequently has a major improvement in their asthma through late childhood, particularly around adolescence in males.

2    Sex of the child
     There is an unexpected difference in the frequency of asthma in boys compared with girls between children and adults. In early childhood, the male to female ratio is approximately two to one. In adulthood, this ratio is virtually reversed. It is now clear that during adolescence (puberty) asthma frequently disappears in males, but frequently appears for the first time in females. The explanation for this remains unknown, but presumably relates to the complex hormonal and growth differences between girls and boys at puberty.

3    The presence of other allergic problems (nasal allergy or eczema)
     Many studies demonstrate a close relationship between disease severity and the presence of other allergic (atopic) problems.
     There are a number of so-called 'birth cohort' studies which have examined children from birth through to mid-childhood. These show a strong association between atopy, either as measured by allergen skin-prick testing or by the presence of clinical atopy (nasal allergy/eczema), and persistence of both asthma and bronchial hyper-responsiveness. These studies suggest that children with wheeze can be classified into two distinct groups:
     First, a 'favourable' group, who commence to wheeze in the first one to two years of life, do not develop atopy (either on skin testing or

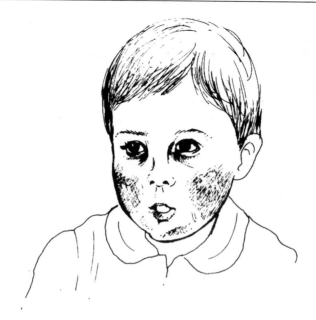

**Figure 10.1**: Child with eczema on face and 'allergic shiners'
(dark circles under eyes)

clinically), and who cease wheezing by school age. In this favourable
sub-group, it has been suggested that the risk for persistent wheezing
(asthma) in mid-childhood (age 10 to 11 years) is approximately 25 per
cent (a one-in-four chance of persistent asthma).

In the 'unfavourable' group, wheezing begins later (over the age of two
years), the children are atopic on skin testing and clinically, and they
have classical asthma in mid to late childhood. The risk of persisting
asthma in this latter sub-group was 80 per cent (four out of five chance
of persistent asthma). Studies such as these allow a statistical probability (risk or odds) to be applied in a given individual child, at an early
age, in an effort to predict the likelihood of subsequent asthma.

4    Allergic family history
If either the child's parents, or siblings have clinical allergy (asthma,
hay fever/nasal allergy or eczema), then the risk of asthma developing
is greater than if these features are not present. Moreover, the risk of
persistence of asthma into mid-late childhood is also greater. This
observation supports the theory that asthma is genetically based.

5    Age of onset of wheezing
Many have believed that very early onset of wheezing was an
unfavourable feature. Research studies do not support this belief –

indeed most suggest the reverse. However, if a given child has very severe symptoms during the first year of his or her *disease,* this is seen as an unfavourable feature, in terms of possible disappearance of asthma.

6    Early respiratory illness

If a child has severe lower respiratory illness in the first two years of life, there is a high risk of developing wheezing and asthma in later childhood. This is particularly so if the early respiratory illness was acute viral bronchiolitis requiring admission to hospital. In some studies, the rate of subsequent asthma in children admitted to hospital with acute viral bronchiolitis in infancy has been as high as 80 to 90 per cent. For those infants with viral bronchiolitis not admitted to hospital, the risk appears to be no higher than that for an unaffected infant. Whether the bronchiolitis causes subsequent asthma is uncertain. It may be that severe bronchiolitis (requiring admission to hospital) is simply more likely in those infants who were destined to be asthmatics.

7    Diet

There is conflicting evidence about the role of prolonged breastfeeding versus artificial feeding in childhood asthma. Recent studies, with better scientific design, do not support the theory that prolonged breastfeeding prevents the development of respiratory atopy (asthma or nasal allergy). However, eczema may be delayed by prolonged breastfeeding. There is also recent evidence suggesting that children who eat fish on a regular basis are less likely to develop asthma: that is, asthma may be prevented. However, eating regular fish meals does *not* influence the course of asthma in those who already have the disease.

8    Passive smoking

There is very strong evidence that exposure to tobacco smoke either before (in utero) or after birth, leads to a greater risk of asthma. The risk appears to be between 1.5 to 2 times the background risk of asthma. There is also evidence indicating that the severity of the disease and, therefore its likelihood to persist, is also influenced by exposure to tobacco smoke. In some studies, this effect is particularly impressive in male children. The major importance of this finding is that exposure to passive smoking is a totally *preventable* risk factor, over which parents have total control.

## CAN ASTHMA BE PREVENTED?

The location of a single gene for asthma and atopy has been recently proposed. Confirmation of this and further characterisation of this gene appears imminent. Intervention programs, that can avoid environmental triggers which operate on

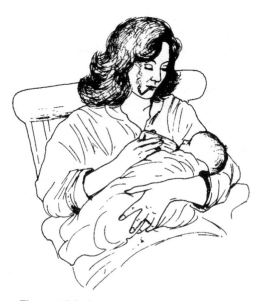

**Figure 10.2:** Passive smoke exposure in infancy

**Table 10.1:** Risk factors for persistence of asthma

| Favourable | Unfavourable | Questionable |
|---|---|---|
| Mild episodic asthma | Severe chronic asthma (especially if severe during first year of disease) | Early, effective medical management |
| Episodes only with viruses | Multiple triggers of attacks | Prolonged breastfeeding |
| Absence of atopic conditions | Other atopic conditions (eczema, nasal allergy) | Regular fish meals |
| Very early onset of wheeze (especially first year of life) | Late onset of wheeze (especially after second year of life) | Air pollution |
| No family history of atopy | A family history of atopy ( parents/siblings) | |
| Persistently negative allergen skin-prick tests (or RAST) | Multiple and/or large positive allergen skin-prick tests (or RAST) | |
| Non-exposure to passive smoking | Exposure to passive smoking before and after birth | |

the genetically susceptible to cause allergic disease (particularly asthma) may then be possible. A popular theory is that the early triggers are respiratory viruses and the common indoor allergen, house dust mite. There may well be an interaction between these two triggers in individual children. While it is impossible to prevent viral infections at present, measures are being developed which could minimise exposure to house dust mite, at least for a short time of the child's life. Thus, it is possible that prevention of exposure to both house dust mite and respiratory viruses in the first months of life could prevent asthma – in at least some of the genetically predisposed children. However, considerably more research is necessary in this area before this theory can be proven.

## THE ADULT WITH ASTHMA

Although asthma may start for the first time in adult life, the majority of adults with asthma will have experienced symptoms of asthma in childhood. A major study of the natural history of asthma from childhood into adult life was carried out in Melbourne. In the late 1960s, school children with asthma were enrolled from seven years of age, and these children were seen at regular intervals through childhood, adolescence and early adulthood. By the age of 14, almost half of these children had ceased wheezing, but when reviewed at the age of 21, many had recurrences of their wheezing. The severity of asthma in childhood was predictive of both the likelihood of ongoing asthma and the severity of asthma at the age of twenty one. That is, those with mild asthma tended to become wheeze-free, or remain mild, while those with severe asthma continued to have persistent symptoms. In fact, less than 20 per cent of those with persistent asthma symptoms in childhood became totally wheeze-free at 21 years of age.

It is a common belief that while asthma is less common in adult life, the disease severity is worse. However, a recent survey of around 9000 primary school children, and their parents, living along the east coast of Australia has cast doubt on this belief. The frequency of recent wheezing (during the past 12 months) was almost 20 per cent for both the children and the adults. While 17.2 per cent of the children had been diagnosed as having asthma, only seven per cent of the adults reported that their respiratory symptoms were diagnosed as asthma.

There are a number of possible reasons for these differences, including a reluctance by adults to visit their doctor for diagnosis, or under diagnosis of asthma by their doctors. These results suggest that there are a similar number of adults and children, having symptoms of asthma (especially wheeze). Further, since the majority of adults with wheeze have not been diagnosed as having asthma, most, presumably, have mild (or trivial) disease. Thus, the prevalence and spectrum of asthma in adults appear to be very similar to that of childhood asthma, as described in this book.

The approach to the treatment of the adult with asthma is very similar to the principles of treatment outlined in the previous chapters. It is hoped that the child and adolescent with asthma will have gained the knowledge about their disease to manage their asthma confidently, in adult life, with appropriate medication and attention to avoidance, or modification of trigger factors.

---

### SUMMARY: WILL MY CHILD GROW OUT OF ASTHMA?

- Although there are many questions yet to be answered regarding the natural history of childhood asthma, a number of markers can be identified which enable a 'risk profile' to be drawn-up for a given individual child.
- This 'risk profile' is similar to the risk profile for adults with respect to cardiovascular disease (heart attacks and strokes) such as high blood pressure, high cholesterol, positive family history, obesity.
- Risk factors associated with an unfavourable prognosis for asthma include: later onset of wheeze; severity of symptoms; a personal or family history of allergy (atopy) and exposure to cigarette smoke.
- It is now a matter of confirming these risk factors, identifying others, and developing methods of reducing these environmental factors.
- It seems certain that this aspect of childhood asthma will be clarified in the near future, particularly if the recent discovery of the proposed atopic gene is confirmed.
- It is becoming clearer that the majority of adult asthma begins in childhood and the prevalence, severity and approach to treatment of adult asthma is similar to childhood asthma.

# 11

# COMMONLY ASKED QUESTIONS AND ANSWERS

---

1   Why are Australians particularly prone to asthma than people in other countries? Are Aborigines at as much risk as white Australians?

The question of differing asthma prevalence in different populations, as well as apparent changes in prevalence over time, is a complex one.

There are a variety of differences which may account for differing prevalence, and these include inherited factors,environmental factors or different criteria for the diagnosis of asthma. It does appear that the prevalence of asthma in Australia and New Zealand is the highest in the world, but the exact reason for this remains unclear.

Asthma does appear to be lower in the Aboriginal race, and is probably related to genetic factors.

2   Is asthma contagious?

No. Asthma is due to a combination of inherited factors, which pre-dispose to the development of asthma, and environmental factors which result in the clinical expression of the disease. Although infections may trigger episodes of wheezing, asthma is *not* an infection and is therefore not contagious.

3   Given the advancements in drugs and treatments, why has the death rate from asthma been increasing?

Although there has been an increase in the death rate for asthma in Australia, this increase has been mainly in two age groups: the adolescent/young adult and the elderly. There has been no change in the childhood death rate (under 14 years). It is also important to realise that the death rate is very low considering the high prevalence of asthma in the community. Fortunately, the most recent mortality figures have shown a decline in mortality, which might suggest that some of the predisposing factors are now being rectified.

Different factors may account for increases in death rates in the different age groups, although some factors such as improved recognition of asthma may account for relative increases at all ages. In the adolescent/ young adult population, under-assessment and under-treatment as a result of denial of disease, and poor compliance with preventive treatment are the two major factors. In the elderly, the increasing life span and presence of co-existent disease are important factors. Over-reliance of bronchodilator medication, without appropriate use of preventive medication, is another factor which has recently been proposed as a possible contributor to the increase in death rate.

**4**  Can children die from asthma? How can I prevent this from happening, especially when I am not with my child?

The death rate from asthma in childhood (under 14 years) is low, accounting for no more than 20 deaths per year in Australia and this rate has not changed significantly over the past 20 years. Generally, children with more severe forms of asthma are most at risk, although rarely, death has been known to occur unexpectedly in apparently mild asthma.

The major ways to prevent death from asthma are to ensure that your child has been appropriately assessed, and treatment prescribed according to his or her severity. You should have a written management plan, including an action plan, to be used in the event of an acute severe episode of wheezing. If the child is prescribed preventive treatment, this should be taken regularly. Bronchodilator medication should be available to your child at all times for treatment of wheezing episodes. When children are old enough, you should encourage them to learn about their disease and allow them, gradually, to take over the responsibility for its management.

**5**  Can children under the age of one get asthma? Are there any particular ages at which children seem to have more problems with asthma?

Wheezing is a common problem in the first year of life, because infants have much smaller airways. The diagnosis of asthma is more difficult to make in this age group as many wheezy infants do not continue to wheeze after the first 12 or 18 months of life. However, some wheezy infants do have more typical asthma symptoms in the first year of life. Asthma is most common in the pre-school age group and is usually related to viral infections such as the common cold. Many of these children appear to improve after the pre-school years. While asthma is less common in the older age groups, there is a relative increase in the more troublesome forms of asthma.

For more details on this question, see Chapter 3: Asthma through the ages.

**6**    At what age do most children 'grow out' of asthma?

It is clear that while many children with asthma improve as they get older, and even appear to lose their tendency to wheeze, they probably retain the potential to wheeze throughout their lives. Many children have reduced symptoms after the pre-school years, while others appear to improve at puberty, but follow-up studies indicate that at least some of those who have apparently 'grown out' of their asthma will wheeze again in adult life. In general, however, if wheezing recurs, the pattern of severity is similar to that during childhood. See Chapter 10 which deals with this question in more detail.

**7**    What information should I tell the teacher or pre-school about my child?

The school should know that your child suffers from asthma: how severe it is; what is likely to trigger wheezing; what treatment the child is having; who the doctor is and his or her phone number. You should demonstrate to the teacher the medication and device your child is using. Ideally you should be able to provide them with a copy of the management plan, including the action plan, for treatment of an acute episode of wheezing. Schools are now being encouraged to involve the teachers in asthma education and to provide bronchodilator medications in their first-aid kits.

**8**    Are there any special things I need to do before going overseas with a child who has asthma?

This will depend on the severity of your child's asthma and the duration of the visit. Things that may need to be considered include: a letter from your doctor outlining the child's drug therapy; an adequate supply of medication; appropriate pump for power supply (if nebuliser needed); and referral to appropriate medical practitioners overseas. Children with asthma will generally have no major problems with air travel, but if their asthma is unstable and they require special treatment during the flight, this will need to be discussed with the airline.

**9**    How do I tell when my child is wheezy? I can never hear anything in his or her chest even when it is obvious that my child is having trouble breathing?

Signs such as how fast your child is breathing, how laboured the breathing is and how active he or she is, may be more useful than hearing a wheeze. Some children with quite audible wheezing may not have any significant breathing difficulty, while others who are clearly distressed with their breathing may not sound wheezy, as there is insufficient movement of air to create a wheezing noise. If the child is old enough to use a peak flow meter, this will give you a more objective assessment of the degree of airway narrowing. In addition, the response to bronchodilator medication in terms of relief of breathing difficulty or improvement in peak flow rate will also be useful.

**10** What signs should we look for to know that our child needs to start on the preventive medications?

A decision regarding the use of preventive medications will depend on the frequency of the episodes of wheezing, and the presence of symptoms between episodes. Details of the assessment of severity in childhood asthma are outlined in Chapter 4 of this book.

**11** When should my child use the peak flow meter?

The use of peak flow monitoring in childhood asthma is discussed in detail in Chapter 4: Assessing Severity. In brief, it is generally inappropriate in children under five years of age as it is likely to be unreliable and is most useful in children with more severe or unstable forms of asthma. However, a period of monitoring may be helpful in the initial assessment of a child with asthma, particularly if there is some doubt about severity. Additionally, it may be useful when stabilising asthma or during reduction in treatment.

**12** How long can I expect my child to have continuing cough and/or wheeze after being discharged from hospital?

This will vary according to the severity of the episode and the pattern of underlying asthma. In general, episodes which require hospitalisation will tend to be more severe than those not requiring hospitalisation, and so symptoms may take several days to resolve completely after discharge. Some children may have a transient increase in their airway sensitivity following such an episode and therefore, tend to have some low-grade symptoms such as cough at night-time or with exercise.

**13** How often should a child be seen by a doctor when he or she has asthma?

This will depend on a number of factors, including the severity and stability of the asthma and the progress on treatment. Your doctor will usually indicate how often an appointment is required, but if you have any worries about your child's asthma, an earlier appointment is appropriate.

**14**    When should I see a specialist as opposed to a general practitioner?

Again, this will depend on the nature and severity of your child's asthma and response to treatment. The usual indications for referral include any unusual symptoms; poor response to treatment or the need for moderate to high-dose inhaled steroid therapy; or frequent courses of oral steroid therapy. You should discuss the need for referral to a specialist with your general practitioner if you have concerns.

**15**    Should I avoid sending my child to day care, especially during winter, as infections are easily picked up and this always provokes the asthma?

Although viral infections are the most common cause of acute episodes of wheezing in childhood, particularly in the pre-school age group, they are difficult to avoid. While avoiding child care may delay the advent of frequent viral infections, it will not prevent them. It is important that the child with asthma has as normal a lifestyle as possible and with appropriate preventive treatment, your child should be able to attend child care, play group and other pre-school activities without problem.

**16**    What measures can we take to reduce the amount of house dust mite, and is this really needed?

The question of house dust mite avoidance is discussed in Chapter 5: Triggers are they avoidable? The need for house dust mite avoidance will depend on whether the child is house dust mite-allergic, the severity of the asthma, and the degree of control of his or her symptoms on conventional therapy. The measures available are outlined in detail in Chapter 5, but current evidence suggests that in Australian conditions, even very strict avoidance measures will not eradicate house dust mite.

**17**    Are there any places suggested not to take a child with asthma?

Again, emphasis should be on trying to achieve a normal lifestyle for the child with appropriate preventive treatment. While it may be prudent to avoid additional triggers during an acute episode of wheezing, when the child is well there is usually no need to restrict outings because of climatic conditions. If the child is known to be sensitive or allergic to certain things, clearly these should be avoided if possible or appropriate preventive treatment given.

**18**    Are some exercises more suitable to keep asthmatics fit than others? For example, swimming.

Exercise-induced asthma and its prevention are discussed in detail in Chapter 5: Trigger Factors: are they avoidable? While swimming is less likely to provoke exercise-induced wheezing than running, with appropriate premedication, a child with asthma should be able to participate in any sport.

**19** How close together can medication (Ventolin) be given if I feel tight in the chest during soccer?

Ventolin can be given safely on a number of occasions during exercise. However, if there is a poor response to treatment or if there is a frequent need for Ventolin, then it is best to stop and rest rather than continuing activity. The need for frequent doses of Ventolin during exercise should serve as an indication to review the regular preventive treatment and the pretreatment regime used *before* exercise.

**20** How will my child's asthma affect our family routine and relationships?

It is important that your child's asthma does not interfere with the normal family relationships. This can be achieved by discussing the nature and treatment of the child's asthma with all members of the family and again ensuring that he or she is treated as normal as possible, albeit with the appropriate use of medication and other preventive measures.

**21** Should I keep on with medications even when my child is not wheezy?

Certain medications are designed to be taken on a regular basis to prevent asthma occurring (preventive medications include Intal and inhaled steroids such as Becotide, Aldecin, Pulmicort) while others are used to treat symptoms of wheezing (relieving medications or bronchodilators). The need for preventive treatment will depend on the asthma severity, but if prescribed, it should be taken regularly. These medications are discussed in detail throughout this book.

**22** How do I know when to reduce my child's asthma medications?

Your doctor will advise you on the use of the different asthma medications in your child. In general, the relieving or bronchodilator medications can be reduced once the wheezing has settled. The preventive medications should be taken regularly, but if your child remains well for some period of time, your doctor may suggest a reduction in dosage.

**23** What are the long-term effects of taking inhaled steroids (Becotide, Aldecin, Pulmicort) for a young child? Do these medications affect their growth?

In general, the potential for side effects with inhaled steroids will depend on the dose used, and how sensitive the child is to the medication. The risk of side-effects with inhaled steroids is much less than with oral steroids as only very small amounts of the inhaled steroid are absorbed into the bloodstream. In addition, they are very effective in controlling children with the more severe forms of asthma. Thus, the

potential for side-effects must be balanced against the potential benefits in individual children. The potential for long-term effects on
growth and other parameters appears to be dependent on dose of medication, severity of asthma and individual susceptibility, and it is only
with further evaluation that these questions will be fully answered.
However, armed with this information of the potential for side-effects,
inhaled steroids can be used appropriately and safely in children with
asthma.

**24**   Can Beconase, nasal steroids and inhaled steroids be given at the same
time? Are there more side-effects when the two are taken together?

Nasal steroids (Beconase, Aldecin, Rhinalar, Rhinocort) used to treat
nasal allergic problems can be combined with inhaled steroids used for
asthma, as often these two conditions co-exist. The risk of additional
side-effects is small, because the dose of nasal steroid required is low.

**25**   Why do some children get less side-effects from Bricanyl than
Ventolin?

Both these medications will tend to make children overactive,
particularly when used in oral or nebulised forms. Individual children
appear to tolerate one medication better than the other, for no apparent
reason.

**26**   Are humidifiers helpful during an asthma attack?

Humidifiers generally have little effect on the lower airways (in the
lung) and provide humidification mainly of the nose. Therefore, they
usually do little during an asthma attack – apart from perhaps helping
to clear nasal secretions.

**27**   How frequently can parents administer Ventolin by way of the
nebuliser at home without going to hospital?

In general, we suggest that if children need the nebuliser more
frequently than every three to four hours, particularly if response is
poor, they require assessment either by their doctor or in the casualty
department of a hospital. As there may be individual differences,
according to the pattern of asthma in your child, this question should be
discussed with your doctor. In general if you are concerned about your
child during an acute episode of wheezing, you should have the child
assessed so that appropriate treatment can be instituted.

# GLOSSARY

---

**Acute severe asthma:** episode of asthma (airway narrowing) which is responding poorly to the child's usual bronchodilator medications.

**Adrenergic system:** that part of the nervous system which opens the airways of the lungs.

**Airway hyper-responsiveness:** increase in the sensitivity of the airway seen in asthmatic patients, which results in the airways narrowing in response to exposure to a variety of trigger factors (viruses, exercise, allergies, and others).

**Airway Inflammation:** changes in the airways of asthmatic patients, characterised by the disruption of the normal cellular lining and accumulation of inflammatory cells (particularly eosinophils). This inflammation is thought to contribute to airway hyper-responsiveness.

**Allergens:** foreign substances ( foods or airborne particles) which lead to the development of antibodies, particularly IgE, which result in 'allergic reactions' on subsequent exposure to that substance.

**Alveoli:** air sacs of the lung which allow exchange of oxygen in the air for carbon dioxide in the bloodstream.

**Anti-cholinergics:** medications which cause relaxation of the muscle around the airway wall by blocking the cholinergic system.

**Atopy:** the tendency to develop allergic (IgE) antibodies following exposure to foreign substances.

**Atopic disease:** those diseases which are associated with atopy, for example, asthma, eczema and allergic nasal symptoms.

**Beta agonists:** medications which relax the muscle around the airway by stimulating the adrenergic system ( Berotec, Bricanyl, Respolin, Ventolin).

**Bronchi:** branching tubes (airways) in the lung which carry air to the air sacs (alveoli).

**Bronchitis:** inflammation of the bronchi, which results in cough and sputum production.

**Bronchiolitis:** inflammation of the smaller bronchi (bronchioles) which is most commonly due to the respiratory syncytial virus (RSV) and results in a wheezing illness in infancy.

**Bronchoconstriction:** narrowing of the airways as a result of contraction of the muscle around the airway wall.

**Bronchodilation:** opening of the airways as a result of relaxation of the muscle around the airway wall.

**Bronchodilators:** medication which result in bronchodilation, for example, Beta agonists, Anti-cholinergics, Theophyllines.

**Chesty child:** a child who is particularly prone to symptoms of cough, wheeze or noisy, 'rattly' chest.

**Cholinergic system:** that part of the nervous system which closes the airways of the lung.

**Co-management:** management involving both the doctor and patient/parent in treatment decisions.

**Cough:** explosive release of air from the chest at high speed for the purpose of removing secretions or irritants from the bronchi and lungs.

**Freon:** liquified gas propellant used in metered dose inhaler (also known as CFCs).

**Hyper-secretory asthma:** form of asthma where mucus production appears to be the predominant pathology and cough the predominant symptom.

**Interval symptoms:** symptoms occurring between the more acute episodes of wheezing, for example, persistent night-time cough, exercise-induced wheezing, morning cough/wheeze.

**Lung function test:** tests which measure the normal function of the lung, that is, moving air in and out of the lungs and exchanging oxygen for carbon dioxide.

**Natural history:** the normal evolution of a disease process, if left untreated.

**Peak Expiratory Flow Rate (PEFR):** measurement of maximal rate of airflow during a forced breathe out after a maximal breathe in. It provides a relatively simple way to measure the presence of airway narrowing in older children and adults.

**Preventers:** medications which, if taken regularly, will prevent episodes of cough and wheeze occurring, for example, disodium cromoglycate (Intal) or inhaled corticosteroids (Becotide, Pulmicort).

**Relievers:** medications which relieve the acute symptoms of asthma by overcoming airway narrowing, for example, bronchodilators, oral corticosteroids.

**Spirometry:** measurement of airflow from a maximum breathe in to a maximum breathe out. It provides a more sensitive measure of airway narrowing than PEFR.

**Trachea:** main airway of the lungs from which the bronchi originate.

**Trigger factors:** those factors which are known to trigger airway narrowing in asthmatic patients, for example, viral infections, exercise, allergies and others.

**Wheeze:** whistling noise arising from the chest, sometimes accompanied by a sensation of difficult breathing.

# Index